"A STRIKING PORTRAIT . . . Employing a journalist's 'fly on the wall' strengths of observation, rendering insights with novelistic verve, Gutkind recounts hospital procedures—from organ transplants to therapy for child-abuse cases—and chronicles a procession of tragedies and triumphs."   —*Publishers Weekly*

"Here are interviews with the gruff dean of transplant surgery, Thomas Starzl; with the astute group of 'pediatricians' pediatricians' who attract interns and residents from all over the country to this hospital; with pumped-up EMS technicians, frustrated social-workers, the designer who brought cheerful pink dinosaurs to the corridor walls, obsessed or merely concerned mothers and fathers, and brave and resilient patients. . . . Best of all are the portraits of doctors and nurses, sometimes heroes, sometimes selfish and spoiled—not gods, but human."   —*Kirkus Reviews*

"Science writer Lee Gutkind examines the roles of health-care professionals and staff, and their relationships with patients and families. He also explores the ethical dilemmas posed by the technological advances of organ transplantation, neonatal life-support, and other medical procedures. . . . Central to the book, however, are the human relationships and emotions experienced on a daily basis."   —*Library Journal*

LEE GUTKIND is the winner of the American Heart Association's Howard W. Blakeslee Award for outstanding achievement in scientific journalism. He is the author of six previous books, including *Many Sleepless Nights: The World of Organ Transplantation*. Lee Gutkind is a professor of English at the University of Pittsburgh and the founder of the university's creative writing workshops for medical professionals.

Other Books by Lee Gutkind

Bike Fever

The Best Seat in Baseball, But You Have to Stand

God's Helicopter (a novel)

The People of Penn's Woods West

Our Roots Grow Deeper Than We Know (an anthology)

Many Sleepless Nights: The World of Organ Transplantation

One Children's Place

A Profile
of Pediatric Medicine

Lee Gutkind

A PLUME BOOK

PLUME
Published by the Penguin Group
Penguin Books USA Inc., 375 Hudson Street, New York, New York 10014, U.S.A.
Penguin Books Ltd, 27 Wrights Lane, London W8 5TZ, England
Penguin Books Australia Ltd, Ringwood, Victoria, Australia
Penguin Books Canada Ltd, 10 Alcorn Avenue, Toronto, Ontario, Canada M4V 3B2
Penguin Books (N.Z.) Ltd, 182–190 Wairau Road, Auckland 10, New Zealand

Penguin Books Ltd, Registered Offices: Harmondsworth, Middlesex, England

Published by Plume, an imprint of New American Library, a division of Penguin
Books USA Inc. This is an authorized reprint of a hardcover edition published by
Grove Weidenfeld.

First Plume Printing, October, 1991
10 9 8 7 6 5 4 3 2 1

 REGISTERED TRADEMARK—MARCA REGISTRADA

LIBRARY OF CONGRESS CATALOGING-IN-PUBLICATION DATA
Gutkind, Lee.
    One Children's Place : a profile of pediatric medicine / Lee
Gutkind.
        p.   cm.
    Reprint. Originally published: New York: Grove Weidenfeld. 1990.
    Includes index.
    ISBN 0-452-26687-4 : $19.95
    1. Children's Hospital of Pittsburgh.   I. Title.
    [DNLM: 1. Children's Hospital of Pittsburgh.   2. Hospitals.
Pediatric—Pennsylvania.   3. Pediatrics.   WS 28 AP4 P6C5G 1990a]
RJ27.3.P4G873   1991
362.1′1′0974886—dc20
DNLM/DLC
for Library of Congress   91-26974
                                                              CIP

Printed in the United States of America

PUBLISHER'S NOTE
In certain cases, pseudonyms have been used to protect patient and family
confidentiality. Everyone who appears in this book is real, however, as are their
stories.

To my partner, Patricia Park,
whose intellectual and emotional support
has always been vital

Acknowledgments

THIS is my fifth nonfiction book. All five focus on the feelings and points of view of people with special interests and concerns. Most of those about whom I have written have been cooperative and patient, but I had never before met a group of people as nice and as honest as those at One Children's Place. I wish to express my sincere appreciation to them, and to others who helped me at the University of Pittsburgh, the American Academy of Pediatrics, the American Board of Pediatrics, and the National Association of Children's Hospitals and Related Institutions (NACHRI), as well as to my transcriptionist, Gary Pletsch.

Contents

Foreword

AFTER devoting the past two years to researching and writing this book, I have come to believe that pediatrics (as compared with surgery, internal medicine, etc.) and the special institutions in which it is practiced—children's hospitals—have not been accorded the attention and respect they deserve. This is not surprising, considering the fact that children in the United States are not accorded the attention and respect they deserve either. Children are our country's most crucial natural resource, yet one in five currently lives below the poverty line. To think that we can send satellites to distant planets or pay athletes millions of dollars a year to swat a baseball, shoot hoops, or endorse shaving products, while we fail to feed and educate properly the generation that will succeed us, is an inexcusable and unjustified irony.

Although they treat only about 10 percent of the sick children in the United States, most frequently those whose lives are in jeopardy, children's hospitals—places designed specifically to respond to the physical and emotional needs of kids—begin to correct that imbalance. And Children's Hospital of Pittsburgh (official address, One Children's Place) is especially distinctive because of its responsiveness to the community it serves.

After being accorded complete access to the inner workings of the institution and all of the 2,000 employees that help it function, I have been extraordinarily impressed with the compassion for all children, including the most helpless and disenfranchised, demonstrated by nurses, pediatricians, surgeons, administrators, social workers, therapists, and other staff members from all levels of the hospital.

But of all the people I have come to know during my time behind the scenes at One Children's Place, it is the families—the mothers and fathers who dedicate themselves unwaveringly to the well-being of their children—who are most memorable. Never have I witnessed such heroism in the face of such heartbreak, such loyalty in the face of such despair. All parents are not good parents or even good people, I have discovered, but mothers and fathers like Debbie and Danny Burdette have demonstrated the deepest meaning of the concept of nobility.

Part I

Tooling Around in OR #7

Chapter 1

MARC ROWE, chief of Surgical Services at Children's Hospital of Pittsburgh, returned home from Boston, where he had been helping to conduct the surgical certification boards for the American Board of Surgery, at about 9:00 P.M. He sprawled on the sofa in his family room and watched two movies on television, periodically participating in a sporadic conversation with his wife. Although he was not on call that evening, he fully expected to be summoned back to the hospital, so he was on edge, unable to halt the galloping adrenaline—that sense of crisis and immediacy that had been with him throughout his surgical life. But as the hours passed, he began to doze, although it was always difficult to sleep soundly when he suspected, from years of experience, that the telephone would ring, that the voice on the other end would tell him about one of his patients who had taken a bad turn, or a Level I trauma—a critically injured child—who needed help. But tonight he was spared the interruption, and he slept for a few hours before waking, dressing quickly, and driving to the hospital through the foggy dawn.

The men's locker room at Children's Hospital is a shadowed and cramped space with lines of hard wooden benches squeezed between rows of metal lockers. There is a small lounge at the far end of the locker room, off a corridor that leads to the operating suite, and as he undressed, Rowe heard voices coming from that lounge, voices he recognized but did not particularly want to hear at that moment.

He pulled on sweat pants, a sweatshirt, and a fairly new pair of running shoes and left the locker room quickly, taking the elevator from 7 down to G, padding softly past the information desk, and breaking out onto Fifth Avenue in a plodding jog.

"Watch, watch, watch your back!" yells a nurse, as a young resident, masked and in surgical scrubs, arms folded at his chest, backs into a tray of instruments spread out carefully on a blue towel.

Though he has only barely touched the tray with his sleeve, the resident, whose name is Joseph Collela, understands that he has contaminated all the instruments on it and that the entire setup must now be replaced. He rolls his eyes, mumbles an embarrassed apology, and takes a couple of steps sideways, trying to find a safe standing spot here in Operating Room 7 on the sixth level at Children's Hospital. He is waiting to assist the attending surgeon, Dr. Rowe, who has yet to arrive in the OR that early morning.

"We won't crucify you this time," says scrub nurse Suzanne Lomire, "but the next time . . . watch out."

Nancy Van Balen, the circulating nurse, responsible for the preparation of instruments and equipment, as well as the source of all surgical supplies before and during the procedure, quickly folds the contaminated instruments into the blue towel on which they were displayed and carries the entire package away. She then returns with another blue towel, folded similarly, which, with its corners unfolded, reveals a previously sterilized set of instruments, ready for use.

"She didn't like those tools anyway," says Sam Smith, a young and newly appointed attending surgeon, born and raised in Arkansas. "Attending" means that Smith is not only on staff at Children's but is also a faculty member, an assistant professor, in the Department of Surgery at the University of Pittsburgh, the institution with which Children's has long been the clinical pediatric affiliate. "Don't worry," he adds. "The first time I was in an operating room, I started picking up the instruments to see what they looked like. You can just imagine what those nurses did to me."

Smith, who had been a pediatric surgical fellow, training in Pittsburgh for the two years prior to his official appointment, had been replaced by Steve Teich, a balding, egg-shaped man of thirty-four, who has momentarily stepped away from the operating table to tape a surgical mask to the bridge of his nose so that it will not slip during the upcoming procedure. All the while, he continues to observe his patient carefully. The little girl has already been put to sleep but has not yet been completely prepared for surgery by the anesthesiologists milling around the table.

Although the name on the patient's chart, which sits on a shelf in a rear corner of the OR, is Chasity Danielle Burdette, her mother, Debbie, has explained that her first name is actually Chastity but the nurses in the tiny West Virginia hospital in which she was born registered the name on the birth certificate incorrectly. It hardly matters, however, for everyone calls her Danielle, "because that's what her father started to do as soon as she was born." Her father's name is Danny.

"Everyone" means not only Danielle's family, friends, and neighbors in St. Albans, West Virginia (population 12,404), but also the hundreds of other people—nurses, doctors, technicians, and administrators, not to mention the many other patients and families in the hospital—who have come into contact with the Burdettes over the years. Danielle and Debbie have lived most of the five years of Danielle's life at Children's Hospital and have come to exemplify the compassion that an institution, no matter how large, can offer families who are socioeconomically disadvantaged. Danielle suffers from Jeune's syndrome, a deformity in which the ribs are short and the chest wall is abnormally small, preventing any expansion of the developing lung.

The Burdettes are also representative of how the miracle and potential of modern medical technology can confuse reality and unmercifully conflict with the very system that makes the technology work. The fact that Danielle Burdette is alive today is the linchpin of the Burdettes' existence; the fact that Danielle could die today—and worse, that she could die any day thereafter, even if this and subsequent surgeries are wholly successful—is a fact that is too bitter for the Burdettes, or almost anyone else in this hospital, including her surgeons, to swallow.

"If we're going into her chest, will we need a bone saw?" Nancy Van Balen asks Teich.

"No, no bone saw," says Teich. He pauses, shakes his head, and indicates with his shoulders and eyes for Nancy to dab the perspiration from his forehead with a towel. "What we actually need is more heat. This is ridiculous," he adds.

"C'mon, Steve, you have to understand," says Suzanne Lomire, "I'm on a diet. This is how I lose my weight."

Keeping the operating room at approximately 80 degrees is actually a way of safeguarding against hypothermia, a real and constant threat in pediatrics, especially with infants and small children. The room thermostat is equipped with an emergency button that will provide an instant increase in heat, while Danielle's back is simultaneously being warmed by an electrically heated water mattress, which can also cool her down if she becomes overheated. Hanging above Danielle are also two "french fry lights" to further enhance her warmth.

"So jack it up some more, why don't you?" says Teich. "Couldn't we all afford to lose a couple of pounds?"

Usually, only one of Children's nine attending surgeons will scrub for each procedure, along with either a resident or a fellow. Often, since Children's is a teaching institution, if a fellow has scrubbed in, he or she will probably do the surgery, supervised by the attending. Except on rare occasions, residents, limited in experience, will do no more than follow suture lines (hold the long tail of the suture out of the way so that it doesn't obscure the area of the next stitch), tie knots, and generally help to expose the surgical field—no cutting. Because of the danger and the potential complications of Danielle's upcoming operation, Teich and Rowe will do the procedure together, with a second attending, Sam Smith, as an emergency backup in case of trouble, and Collela assisting.

"So Dr. Rowe was up in Boston yesterday playing God?" says Teich.

Unlike most specialties in the field of surgery, which has in general experienced a glut of personnel, pediatrics is a field in which surgeons have long monitored their own growth. Annually, there are in the entire United States only twenty or so pediatric surgical fellowships—the mandatory training position that a doctor must hold in order to be examined for certification by the American Board of Surgery. Although he works 80 to 90 hours a week at Children's, once his fellowship is completed and he passes his boards, an examination similar to, but even more intense than, the bar examination for attorneys, Teich will be virtually assured of a job. In fact, each week he receives an average of three letters inviting him to interview for available positions.

"When I took my surgical boards," says Smith, "it was the scariest day of my life. There you are, facing three hard-assed surgeons, grilling you for hours, who can blow you out of the water with a failing grade after you've dedicated seven years of your life to the field. They'll flunk you if you are late or if you go to the wrong room. I remember going to the room where my examination was scheduled and knocking on the door and no one answered. I knocked a second and a third time—and still no answer. Suddenly I thought I had somehow gone to the wrong room, that my career was over, just like that. Finally, the door opened and this guy was saying, 'Dr. Smith?'

"I said, 'Yes. Am I in the right place?'

"He said, 'Sure, but we were involved in a conversation and just got carried away. Sorry you had to wait.'

"I swear to God," said Smith, "waiting outside that door, I thought I was going to have a heart attack."

Smith dabs Danielle's abdominal area with Betadine and then begins to hook up a Foley catheter for draining urine output. The catheter will also demonstrate how efficiently Danielle's kidneys are functioning during the procedure, with units of fluid per hour computed and flashed on the monitor above the operating table. In addition to the Foley, a blue tube protrudes from her belly, a gastrostomy. "That's how she's fed," says Smith. "Danielle never liked to eat."

The anesthesiologists have also added a tangled mass of wires and alarms to her body. An intravenous (IV) tube has been placed in the vein of her right hand for the admission of blood and other fluids. An oximeter, a little instrument that makes her tiny thumb glow red, measures pulse rate and oxygen in the blood. There's an automatic blood pressure pump on her right arm that prints both systolic (when the heart is pumping) and diastolic (when the heart is relaxing) measurements on the monitor, along with a Broviac catheter, a more permanent type of entryway, or IV, for an influx of medications. Exiting from her mouth is an esophageal stethoscope plugged directly into the anesthesiologist's ear. "You never trust the alarms completely," says Smith. "We want to monitor her breathing continuously."

As he works, Smith tells me that he is very happy to meet a writer and that, in fact, there are many people at Children's interested in literature. "But we usually hide our books from one another. People in hospitals often don't share their private thoughts. It's a cold place sometimes. So many terrible things happen that you normally don't allow yourself to get intimate with or interested in any of the people you work with." He remembers feeling embarrassed and uncomfortable about bringing his guitar to his first Department of Surgery Christmas party, and then discovering three others with guitars.

Before entering the operating room, surgeons scrub at a Fleximatic scrub sink, located in a small windowed room directly adjacent to the OR. Each of two stainless-steel basins is equipped with two hook-shaped, high-necked spouts. Faucets opposite each spout give surgeons a choice of a range of water temperatures, but they are controlled so that surgeons cannot accidentally scald their hands. There are also two stainless-steel boxes below each basin so that soap and water can be activated by knee.

Scrubbing is a therapeutic, even a spiritual experience for most surgeons, perhaps especially Marc Rowe, who quotes frequently from a tiny book called *Zen in the Art of Archery*. The author, Eugen Herrigel, a German philosopher who went to Japan in the 1930s to take up the practice of archery toward an understanding of Zen, writes about the importance of the many customs of preparation— the "meditative repose" in acquiring "that collectiveness and presence of mind without which no right work can be done." Scrubbing is emotionally and intellectually soothing, and it begins for the surgeon that process by which the irreplaceable tools of his trade— the hands and fingers—become first cleansed and then integrated with the mind. After about ten minutes of solitary scrubbing, using a collection of brushes, a fingernail pick, and great quantities of yellow odorless soap, Marc Rowe, fifty-eight, dressed in blue scrubs, with blue paper covers over his running shoes, backs into the operating room, pushing the door with his neck and shoulders, and holding his hands in the air, ready to be gowned and gloved by the waiting nurse.

In contrast to most of his colleagues in surgery, which is typically an upper-middle-class profession, Rowe, a one-time merchant seaman, is deeply rooted in the working class. He has long identified with the disadvantaged, the underdog, in American society, and enjoys telling the story about how he suddenly decided, in his senior year of high school, that he might like to go to college, and how he went to his high school guidance counselor about scholarship opportunities and applications.

"A few days later, one night after dinner, there was a knock on our front door. I was up in my bedroom, and I went out in the hallway to see who it was. It was one of my teachers, who had come to tell my parents, both blue-collar workers, in a polite and embarrassed manner, that their son's sudden interest in college was unrealistic and ill-advised, and that I was intellectually limited, and that I would do much better in life if I took up a trade. In fact, my father was so impressed with this advice that he enrolled me in welders' school following my graduation." A last-minute reprieve came when Rowe won the state high school middleweight wrestling championship in an upset match that earned him a scholarship from Brown University.

Much of his attitude and approach to life and medicine today stems from his experiences as a wrestler and gymnast. "You watch guys who work together on a trapeze. One guy is the swinger and the other guy is the catcher. At a certain point, a swinger has got to let himself go, and throw himself off the trapeze with every bit of abandon he can muster. If he has any lack of courage or of confidence, if he lingers on there just a split second longer, he'll miss the catcher." That, said Rowe, is how to approach highly complicated and difficult surgery. "Once you decide you're going to do it, you just have to throw everything you've got into it, no holds barred, and zingo, that's it. You gotta go all out."

Of late, Rowe has become a marathon runner. "I once was running in the Orange Bowl marathon, and I came up on some guy, and he looked to be in very bad shape, and I ran beside him and I said, 'Are you all right?'

"He said, 'Yes, I'm all right.'

"I said, 'You don't look all right.'

"He said, 'The only way anybody is going to get me to stop is if they shoot me. Because,' he said, 'I'm going to finish this son-of-a-bitching race.'

"Well, it's the same thing in surgery. It's not worthwhile to just do it half way. If you're not going to try to win, there's no sense in doing it at all. But I'm realistic enough to know that you don't always win no matter how hard you try."

Despite his success as a surgeon and many international honors and awards, Rowe remains a product of his past. He is a nondescript man of medium height, with the traditional broad shoulders and barrel chest of the wrestler, as well as the "cauliflower" ears. Those ears, combined with an abrupt and confrontational manner, which many of his pediatrician colleagues at Children's call "downright nasty," are clear-cut and intimidating evidence to anyone who meets him that this man is ready and willing to go to the mat, not only in the surgical and athletic arenas but also in life. His manner is punctuated by a thick New England accent and an irrepressible tendency to use four-letter words, for which he is always apologizing to his women colleagues at Children's.

Both the parents he serves and his colleagues—nurses and doctors alike—say that one of Marc Rowe's strong points is his spontaneous sense of humor, but his moods are so intense and unpredictable that you often never know how to respond to even the most obvious of his actions.

"When we first came up here in October, and I met Dr. Rowe, I thought to myself: He has to be the most arrogant, sarcastic bastard I've met in my life," says Trish Cambron of Kentucky. Trish has been commuting back and forth to Children's with her adopted son, Joshua, who has been under Rowe's care for more than two years. Cambron discovered Joshua in Korea, languishing with an allegedly incurable disease in a tiny orphanage. Rowe saved Joshua's life. "But I would ask Dr. Rowe questions, and he would just keep walking, and wouldn't turn around and answer me, and I would just think: What is it? What? I just want to talk. I just want to know about my child. Every time I would see him, I would feel like I could just cry. I was always afraid he was going to bite my head off."

Trish Cambron remembers waiting once for Rowe to come to report to her after operating on Joshua. She waited for hours in Joshua's room because he had promised to come directly after the procedure was completed. Every time the nurses in the operating room would report to her that he was on the way up to the unit, some problem with another patient would suddenly arise to delay him. But finally the phone rang, and in a deep and threatening voice, Rowe said, "I want to see you in my office right away."

Cambron thought something terrible had happened to Joshua, because she knew that the child was still in the recovery room and because, with the exception of the first visit, Rowe would always meet her in Joshua's room on 9 South, the surgical unit in the hospital. Although she was on the ninth floor, she was too petrified to waste time waiting for the elevator. She ran down five flights of stairs, then down the corridor and into the Department of Surgery. Rowe was waiting at the door. "Get in here; get in my office right away," Rowe said. She rushed in, and he looked at her, paused dramatically, and then, after what seemed an eternity, finally smiled and said, "What took you so long?" All he had wanted to do was talk to her in private, but he had scared her half to death.

"Dr. Rowe has an interesting sense of humor," says Trish Cambron. "Sometimes we have fun together; sometimes we don't."

One of the anesthesiologists has been attempting to sink an A line, or arterial line, into Danielle's foot, in order to have a direct means of measuring oxygen content and blood pressure during surgery. But she seems unable to thread the catheter into the lumen—the space within an artery or vein—a common problem in pediatrics, especially with infants and young children. A tiny pool of blood has now accumulated below Danielle's foot.

As soon as he notices, Rowe immediately informs the doctor that he doesn't think they'll need the arterial line. But the anesthesiologist says that she would feel safer with it in, and she begins listing the reasons that the extra monitoring capacity would be appropriate. Rowe listens, but it is clear from the beginning he is not going to give in. "With a child this ill," he reasons, "you have to safeguard each entryway. You never know when an IV will be necessary either today or sometime in the future. Look," he adds, "I've known this kid for a long time."

The discussion continues back and forth for another five minutes, and although Rowe tries to be diplomatic by telling the anesthesiologist that the final decision is actually hers to make, it is clear that she, as a junior faculty member, is not going to butt heads with the chief of Surgical Services for very long. The topic is permanently put to rest when the pager hooked to the drawstring at the waist of her scrubs begins beeping; she heads for a telephone to answer. The subject of the A line does not come up again.

Rowe steps back behind the table and extends his hands to allow Nancy to snap on his translucent latex gloves. The gowns are awkward; they wrap around you like generous strips of cloth wrapped around mummies. With his hands in the air, cupped into each other, his elbows tight against his ribs, Rowe turns a complete circle as Nancy ties the gown with strings around his back.

A nurse who works for the orthopedic surgeons at Children's, whom Rowe has recruited to participate in this operation, now shows him an array of metal rods of different diameters. Rowe lifts each rod in his gloved hand and examines the thickness under the light before choosing one.

"Do your guys have a regular flat file?"

"No, I don't think so," says the nurse.

"Well, you might get me one from Maintenance."

"Are you serious?" she says.

"Of course I'm serious."

"This sounds more like the motor pool than the operating room."

"To be perfectly honest," says Rowe, "I'm just making this up as I go along. Nothing's ever been done like this before."

Now Marc Rowe turns to the operating table and begins to concentrate on his patient. Rowe points a gloved finger toward her chest, right at the point where he will cut. He examines the stent, a piece of molded plastic shaped like a cork, recently inserted by ENT (ear, nose, and throat) surgeons in order to facilitate Danielle's breathing. During a sudden sickness of undetermined origin (suspected to be some sort of viral pneumonia), which nearly cost her her life, Danielle lost her normal reflexive abilities to dispense with accumulated secretions—saliva and mucus. Her larynx (located at the upper end of the trachea, below the root of the tongue) was opened and plugged with the stent to decrease the possibility of choking and suffocating, thus enhancing the importance of her tracheostomy, which became her only means of breathing. At home or in the Respiratory Care Unit (RCU), where Danielle is often lodged, constant attention must be paid to this last remaining air passage, which could easily become clogged and cause her death.

Rowe is concerned with the stent, not necessarily for the procedure today but because it has not been working effectively and often becomes infected, necessitating more surgery. This is Danielle's third stent in less than a year, with a fourth scheduled sometime in the next few weeks, pending the outcome of today's procedure. The insertion of the stent was not vital. The larynx (the voice box) could have been eliminated entirely (through a laryngectomy), decreasing the likelihood of many complications, but Danielle's mother was unwilling to add lack of speech to Danielle's other disabilities—at least until it became a last resort. With the stent in, Danielle cannot talk, but if her normal reflexes somehow return (she learns to swallow), the stent can be removed and the trachea reconnected. Pending other complications, such as infection or excessive scar tissue, Danielle might then regain her voice. There is a cherry-sized lump caused by the stent at the base of the throat.

Danielle is an unusual-looking child, dark and exotic with subtly unbalanced features, primarily because of a lack of uniform growth. Her head seems a little too large for her tiny, frail frame.

But at the same time, Danielle is also an incredibly charismatic child, with bright eyes and a broad smile that, despite untold pain and suffering, seems impossible to repress. Danielle's long presence at Children's and her upbeat personality make her attractive to personnel throughout the hospital, who would often, on their own time and for no particular reason, visit her. Because she has hardly ever spent time with children her age, she possesses a special ability to relate to adults.

Rowe cups his gloved hands together the way surgeons will do to protect them from contamination, turns his back to his colleagues, and moves momentarily off into a corner. In his long surgical gown, and with his hands cupped and poised, chest-high, it is not difficult to imagine that he is saying a prayer.

Despite his interest in Zen, Rowe is not a religious man, but it has always seemed to me that serious surgery is reminiscent of the religious experience. The surgical gown can be compared to the clergy's robes; the ritual of preparation is as traditional as the ritual and preparation for the highest of holy days. There is hardly a more important day in the life of an average person than the day he or she, or a close friend or family member, goes under the knife. The wielder of that knife, surrounded by his apostles, can give life or take it away. During the procedure, family that have had differences will often come together, cloaking themselves in prayer. Among the people waiting for the outcome, there exists an irreplaceable, albeit temporary, feeling of brotherhood and communion. Surgery, especially that which is not routine, such as the challenge confronting Marc Rowe, Sam Smith, and Steve Teich at this moment, takes place in the fragile and unpredictable church of life and death.

Now, as if some secret sign has passed between the participants, Rowe turns back to the patient on the operating table. The room suddenly grows quiet, while the pace of the activity significantly increases. Collela begins to soak Danielle's chest with Betadine. A nurse slips "surgical telescopes"—little opera glasses often called "loops," which magnify the surgical field by three times, mounted on top of his regular prescription lenses over Rowe's nose. Teich, also wearing "loops," has previously placed a yellow plastic drape over Danielle's chest, and folded a series of blue towels around the drape, concealing every part of Danielle, including her face, except for the area of the chest on which they will do the procedure.

This, in many ways, is the key to the impersonalization of the surgical experience: the fact that the surgical field has no face, voice, or personality and the total and intense focus of a surgeon's attention is a mere square of blood, flesh, and bone. Perhaps it is difficult for some people to imagine that the surgeon can divorce himself from feelings or familiarity with the patient, but it is a necessity that cannot be avoided. Surgery is a very mechanical exercise that requires a thorough knowledge of the anatomy, an ability to follow a long-established and uniform regimentation of procedure, and totally spontaneous courage, instinct, and skill. This rare combination breeds a special confidence, necessary when one human being is going to cut into another—and also, frequently, an intolerably inflated ego, a feeling almost of omnipotence.

In describing this feeling and the personal destruction it can sometimes cause, Rowe refers to a particularly tragic scene in the film *The Great Santini,* in which the father, who has been defeated one evening by his son in a bitterly contested game of one-on-one basketball, practices in the rain the rest of the night in order to beat his boy the following afternoon. "That's the epitome of surgery," says Rowe. "That is precisely who we are. We sometimes cannot conceive of middle age, bad luck, or defeat"—the attitude of choice in OR #7 on this particular morning or perhaps in any operating arena, anytime.

"Okay," says Rowe. "From this point onward, all we are going to talk about is business." He takes a marker and draws a line on the yellow plastic.

"Are you all right?" says Rowe, softly, to no one in particular. "Is everybody all right?" he asks, much louder.

No one acknowledges the question.

"We're going to go now," says Teich, in a voice that quavers ever so slightly.

"So," says Rowe. "Let's begin."

Chapter 2

A STRANGER passing Debbie Burdette in the elevator, the cafeteria, or the waiting room of the Intensive Care Unit at Children's Hospital will see a tall, gangly woman with long dark hair, straight and smooth and hanging down below her shoulders, and very sharp, angular features. She will move quickly, purposefully, looking straight ahead, as if she were on a mission, with a stern and frozen expression of anger and dread on her face.

But this, you soon realize, is her mask—her way of warning people that she may be young and inexperienced but she is not one to be trifled with, especially under this extended biomedical umbrella, an atmosphere she knows better than her own home. She has lived, off and on, in siege at least twenty hours of each twenty-four-hour day in either the Intensive Care Unit or the Respiratory Care Unit at Children's Hospital of Pittsburgh for more than three years—holidays and weekends included. She has seen her only daughter on the brink of death literally dozens of times, and she has seen other mothers and fathers lose their children in less dangerous circumstances more often than she cares to remember. She is a true veteran of this high-acuity pediatric institution, for she was only nineteen years old when it all started. You can recognize the youth and innocence remaining within her during those infrequent moments when she decides to crack a smile. Debbie Burdette's smile can be likened to a rainbow; it sort of appears, makes its wondrous point, and is folded back behind her mask of wariness.

When her daughter was born, the doctors told Debbie and Danny Burdette that Chasity Danielle would die within six hours. "So we waited and waited—and nothing happened," says Debbie matter-of-factly, in a flat voice with the bare echo of a rural lilt. Two weeks later, Danielle contracted pneumonia. Once again, the doctors said that her death was imminent, and once again, after two more weeks, Danielle had somehow managed to stay alive. Throughout this initial ordeal, Danielle's doctors insisted that they could not help the child. Her problem, Jeune's syndrome, is extremely rare.

"More technically, they called it asphyxiating thoracic dystrophy," said Debbie, "but that one word 'thoracic' sort of stuck in my head, even though at first I didn't know what it meant. I got a phone book and looked under chest specialists, and this one doctor, he had the word 'thoracic' under his name, so I thought, 'This is the fellow I'm looking for.' I figured he could fix her up at the hospital and send her home.

"Well, he went over to the hospital, looked at her, and called me back. He said there was nothing he could do, but for me to just hang on, he would try to find somebody who would. That's when he called Dr. Rowe, who called me and said I could bring her out. Dr. Rowe didn't give me any guarantees; he was always straight, right from the beginning. He said, 'You know, pneumonia could eventually kill her, or she could have an operation to prolong her life and in the process she could die with that, too, but you just can't give up on her.' "

Rowe and many of the doctors, nurses, and staff remember Debbie Burdette when she first arrived at Children's in the spring of 1984 because she was so deathly afraid, not only of the machinery and the people at the hospital with their forbidding white coats and blue scrubs and photo identification badges, but of the entire city. Debbie remained petrified of the world outside the hospital for months. "I was a big chicken. I was afraid to go to restaurants, take a bus to Ronald McDonald [a community-sponsored residential facility for families of children in long-term care], walk outside on the streets; I couldn't look people in the eye. It was a shock to me. I left home thinking I would be back in my own bed the day after tomorrow, and two years later, I was still here."

Over that period, Rowe began the painstaking process of splitting Danielle's sternum and enlarging her rib cage. Initially, he inserted plastic plates, which after a short time were replaced by adult ribs, procured from a bone bank in Florida. These procedures were dangerous surgically and took a long time to heal. Danielle was also extremely susceptible to "blue spells," in which breathing becomes difficult, and constant bouts of pneumonia, further inhibiting her ability to breathe and endangering her life. Eventually Danielle was put on a ventilator to support her breathing. She subsequently received a tracheostomy so that the ventilator could be connected to her throat, enabling her to speak somewhat normally and providing a significant amount of mobility. Most recently came the dreaded stents, which have caused a great many bacterial complications.

It would be impossible for Deborah Burdette to count or recount even the majority of the situations that threatened Danielle's life over the long siege of surgeries and the resulting complications, for one can become numb to memory after repeated suffering. For a parent of a child who is chronically and dangerously ill, it is never just one problem plaguing the child but an ever-increasing series of related problems—problems that often seem to surface at the most inconvenient and unpredictable times.

Debbie's husband, Danny, commuted most weekends, sometimes bringing other members of the family, but essentially Debbie was alone with her baby for the whole two years. And even though, for the following year and a half, through Danielle's third and fourth birthdays, they lived basically at home, the Burdettes frequently had to return to Pittsburgh. "The bones Dr. Rowe had put in had started to deteriorate, so he had to put some more plastic in. And then he put wires in to keep the plastic in, and they came through the skin. He fixed the wires, and then we saw this other piece of plastic coming through the skin, so then he had to go back and fix that."

Rowe could not then and cannot now speculate about how often such instances will occur, but he does know that more procedures will be necessary as Danielle grows older. Even now, in OR #7, attempting once again to widen the chest so that Danielle's lungs will be provided with more room to grow and breathe, he is not certain whether this operation will be enough to permit her to function—even temporarily. "Lots of times, a surgeon's work depends on the patient, his or her will to live," said Rowe. "Some sick kids just roll over and die, while other kids you can't kill with a stick." Rowe and others have speculated that much of Danielle's will to live has come from the will of her mother, who refused to capitulate to what everyone said was inevitable, despite her own vulnerability.

"The first time I arranged for Debbie to go out to the Ronald McDonald House," said Wes Weidenhamer, then the social worker assigned to the Burdettes' case, today vice president of marketing and medical relations at Children's, "she was a terrified little girl from the backwoods of West Virginia. I said to Debbie, 'Look, I've arranged for you to go to the Ronald McDonald House so you can sleep. And I will take you out there.' Well, I could see the fear and trepidation in her eyes as she clutched her suitcase." With Weidenhamer's help, the Burdettes were able to declare permanent residency at the McDonald House, qualifying them for Pennsylvania medical assistance. "West Virginia would not pay because they thought that Danielle's surgery was experimental."

Although Weidenhamer is no longer a social worker, he has maintained contact with Debbie Burdette over the years, often making the facilities of his office—especially his long-distance telephone—available to her. "So it costs a couple of bucks for her to call her mom or call her husband, but this hospital is a community resource. It's the least we can do, although I'm sure there are people who would disagree with that."

Back then, it was not only the social workers but also the surgeons and the pediatricians at Children's who would find themselves working harder for the Burdettes, simply because Debbie seemed so young and vulnerable, so innocently trusting. This situation hasn't changed for the physicians, or the entire medical and administrative staff, who will dote on Debbie and Danielle to an incredible degree. Danielle's photo as a two-year-old, subtly supported by a ventilator, is used as an illustration in the Children's Hospital Directory of Services and on the cover of a brochure describing the facilities of the Respiratory Care Unit. When visitors—possible funding sources and/or legislators with special interests in health care—come to the hospital, Debbie and Danielle are often obligatory first stops. In fact, it was Pennsylvania Republican senior Senator John Heinz, a member of the Children's Hospital Board of Trustees, who pledged to Debbie Burdette on television that Medicare coverage to support Danielle's surgeries, her ventilator dependency, and her home nursing care would continue without interruption, despite threats by the government to the contrary. Weidenhamer has become so attached to Debbie and Danielle that he continues to carry Danielle's 1984 blue plastic treatment card (similar to a charge card) in his wallet as a good-luck charm.

As time has passed, Debbie Burdette has become—for the sake of her child's life—quite capable in the art and science of fighting with or manipulating the people who have attempted to support her so paternalistically. Not that she is ungrateful or that she suspects ill will—on the contrary—but she has come to realize that the world is populated with many well-meaning people with a multitude of conflicting agendas.

She remembers first confronting Rowe about nagging problems concerning Danielle's long-term care after Danielle had had two chest surgeries and had been trached and a gastrostomy tube had been inserted. The trach has always caused a great deal of infection and discomfort for Danielle. The nurses, perfectly correct in their assessment of the ill-fitting trach, had repeatedly mentioned the problem to Rowe, who took no action, and so they urged Debbie to take the matter in her own hands.

"He walked in one day, and I said, 'What are you going to do about this trach?'

" 'Just what do you mean, What am I going to do with this trach?' Dr. Rowe said.

" 'Well, look at it. It's ugly for one thing; it's dirty; it's too small; it's just a mess.' I went on and on, and everyone in that room just stopped to look." No one, apparently, had the courage to talk to Marc Rowe like that.

"He said, 'I've been doing trachs for fifteen years, and you're going to tell me how to do this? I was probably one of the men who invented these things, and you're going to tell me?'

"He said, 'I think you've been listening to these nurses; they don't have the guts to say what you just said. If they have a question, you tell them to come and ask me.' "

"Look, Debbie," said Rowe, trying to indicate his understanding, "we're friends, and we've always been friends, and if you want to continue to be friends . . ."

"I really wanted to sit there and bawl my eyes out," Debbie says, but after that confrontation, "I wouldn't allow myself to shed a tear, even if he cussed me for hours."

From that point on, she was a different person toward doctors and nurses alike. "I just sat down after that experience and realized that Danielle can't speak up, so somebody has to. So if I feel something's wrong, it's got to be me to speak up about it, I guess. My husband doesn't say much; he says I say it all."

One evening recently, a nurse began to refer to three children on the opposite end of the Respiratory Care Unit, where Danielle

Burdette is located, as "the Supremes," probably because they had been there, side by side, for a long period of time. The children were unable to exert control of their bodily functions, and because of her encephalopathy (a dysfunction of the brain contracted during a recent severe sickness), Danielle was also frequently spitting up, making a mess. "Anyway, we were all standing around and she—the nurse—said, 'Danielle, you ought to be over there in the corner with the Supremes.'

"Well, I said, 'I don't think so,' and I kind of left it at that.

"My husband got this real white look on his face. I don't think he was sure what I was going to do. But I kind of let that one go. Then she came back a few seconds later and she said, 'Those kids are gross.'

"And I said, 'Isn't your job here to keep those kids from being gross?'

"Then I just had to get out of there because I was going to rip her hair out, strand by strand. So I went downstairs to the cafeteria, and my husband came down later, and I thought he was going to say, 'You should have never said that.' But he was laughing. I said, 'What do you think is so funny?'

"And he said, 'Well, I was watching and just wondering when you were going to put her in her place. You sure did it.'

"But that wasn't the real issue," said Deborah Burdette. "Those were kids, and this was my daughter that nurse was talking about. I went to Therese [the assistant head nurse] about it, and she kind of took care of it." Debbie had asked that this nurse not be assigned to Danielle again.

"And then a few weeks later, for some reason, the same nurse was suddenly back with Danielle. So," said Debbie, "I did not return to Ronald McDonald that night; I stayed all night and took care of my own child. The nurse couldn't touch her.

"So Therese came over to me the following morning, and she said, 'If this nurse is assigned to Danielle tonight, then I suppose you're going to stay again?'

"I said, 'Yes. I think that me and her just are not able to get along. I will stay here indefinitely.'

"So the point was made—finally. But I was ready to stay on that floor with Danielle for the next six months in order to make sure that nurse never went near my daughter again.

"Overall, the nurses do a wonderful job taking care of the kids," says Debbie. "But I think sometimes they don't take a parent's feelings into enough consideration.

"I remember this nurse when Danielle was just a tiny baby, and every time Danielle would go into surgery and come back out, this nurse would always have her cleaned up, have her hair fixed. She would do her nails and everything—I mean, she would polish them. You knew Danielle was sick and she just came out of surgery, but she didn't look it after that nurse took care of her. That was always important to me.

"As far as I am concerned, the nurses don't need to touch her. I'll do for Danielle what she needs, just as I been doing for her whole life. But if the nurses want to take care of Danielle, that's okay with me. But I'll tell you one thing. It may be over my dead body, but they goddam better do it right."

Chapter 3

WITH a stainless-steel scalpel glittering in the overhead light, Marc Rowe follows the guideline he drew with his marker, leaving a thin red line of blood, five inches long, in his wake. Steve Teich lifts a layer of Danielle's skin with retractors while Rowe switches to the Bovie, an electric needle, also known to surgeons as a "firestick," because it simultaneously cuts and cauterizes. First comes a sound similar to a dentist's drill, as the Bovie is being activated, then a slight wisp of smoke, followed by the aroma of singed flesh. Newcomers to surgery find this latter sensation almost unbearable. You have braced yourself for some cutting and perhaps a fair amount of blood, but the sweet and sudden fragrance that accompanies "first cut" will often cause nausea. As Teich and Rowe work, Suzanne moves in and out of the surgical field with the suctioning device, eliminating excess blood.

Neither Rowe nor Teich can be described as particularly graceful as surgeons, but perhaps grace is something that can only be expressed with broad and sweeping gestures, sometimes more easily achievable in adult procedures. Pediatric surgery is necessarily a confining endeavor, simply because the patient is so small and delicate. I am impressed by their dogged and spontaneous precision: tiny, concentrated movements, conservative and careful but steady and assured; no tentativeness represented in their work, even when they reach the chest wall.

"Give me a knife, a real sharp one," says Rowe.

"New blade," says Suzanne. She hands it to Rowe, rather than slapping it into his palm, as those who watch television might expect. Contrary to common belief, most surgeons appreciate a relaxed and informal atmosphere in the operating arena, an atmosphere that seems to enhance rather than retard efficiency. By-the-book procedure often creates exhausting and potentially harmful stress in a situation that, at its best, is fraught with emotional and physical tension. This is not to say that surgeons do not have temper tantrums when the going gets rough; some of the most polite and dignified figures in medical science are known to use unforgivably abusive language to nurses, students, and junior faculty. Even violence is not unheard of. One surgical fellow witnessed a scene in which a resident who had made a serious but not fatal error was grabbed at the shoulders by a senior surgeon and butted in the head.

"Now let's everybody hold still," says Rowe as he cuts into the wall of bone and plastic. "Take a deep breath."

There is a long silence as Rowe works his way through the chest. "Look," says Rowe, "two years ago, I put in plastic struts to push the chest out so that she could breathe more easily, but the chest wall has grown right underneath them." Rowe proceeds to retrieve five white plastic struts varying between one and two-and-a-half inches long, each approximately a half-inch wide. He lines them up on his hand from fingertip to palm. "See this? This is fascinating. I made holes in these struts, and over the months the tissue has grown right into them."

Smith, who had left the OR to retrieve Teich's camera from his office, has now returned. Perched on a "standing stool," often used by observers to peer over a surgeon's shoulders, he snaps a couple of photos of the blood-stained plastic struts.

"Now this is a chance for my hands to get famous," says Collela, as Smith's flash goes off a half dozen times. Collela has assumed responsibility for suctioning. Smith also takes a shot of the white patch of Gortex Rowe had used as a replacement for the pleura, the natural lining between the chest wall and the lung.

With the photo session completed, Rowe and Teich continue to work doggedly, removing all leftover bits of synthetic materials and the thick scar tissue created from previous surgery, while gradually widening the chest to provide Danielle's lungs with as much space as possible in which to breathe and to grow. As he works, Rowe, who seems to have put himself in kind of a trance, oblivious to conversations or activities in the OR around him, periodically mumbles absentmindedly to himself and/or to Teich and Suzanne: "I have no idea what we're doing." After repeating this statement a half dozen times, he suddenly looks up and drops his instruments. He grabs a piece of cardboard from the scrub nurse's waste table, places it on top of Danielle's little belly, picks up his marker, and says, "Now let's draw a picture of what's going to happen next."

Listening to the radio and waiting as the surgeons complete their conference, I ask Nancy about the kind of music the surgeons like. "Everybody always asks me if surgeons prefer opera or jazz or country western while they're operating," she replies. "But the truth is, most surgeons don't care about music one way or the other—the nurses do. We can listen to anything we want, as long as it's low. You want to make a surgeon angry, just blast the radio. They'll hit the roof."

Danielle was anesthetized at 7:15 A.M.; Rowe entered the operating room some two hours later; it is now 12:20 P.M. From time to time, other surgeons will stop in to observe and spend a few minutes passing the time of day, talking almost exclusively about surgery— new procedures, creative ideas, telling old war stories of procedures past—as men in bars will often discuss and debate sports. Each time I observe surgery, I am struck by how much of a macho world the operating theater is and how difficult it must be for a woman surgeon to break into this men's club and find a comfortable place for herself.

There have been few women training for certification in pediatrics at Children's, although the newest "attending" faculty member appointed jointly by the Department of Surgery and Pitt not long ago is Suzanne Ildstad, who considers the women one generation preceding her—physicians who are now Marc Rowe's age—the real pioneers. "The Chief of Surgical Services at Harvard, prior to my residency there, had been quoted as saying that he would never train a woman; that it would be a waste of resources. Other colleagues at Harvard insisted that they would never let a woman join the Massachusetts Medical Society."

By the time Ildstad arrived at Harvard in 1978, there was a new chief of surgery. "So I was the seventh woman to go through the program. In a way, surgery is a very conservative field, and it's been one of the last of the medical specialties to accept women and to treat them as if they belonged. Now there are enough women in surgery that it's not that unusual anymore. I can't even remember recently having families or patients be concerned that I'm female."

It is possible that women find certain surgical challenges easier than do men because of the smaller size of their hands and the fact that "we grew up sewing and knitting," but Ildstad feels that the real measure of success in surgery is not technique but judgment. "It's much easier to do the operation, whatever it is, than to choose the right operation in the first place. That's the real gift of surgery," she says—a gift that Rowe and his colleagues are at this moment attempting to demonstrate as they labor in OR #7. Utilizing a tiny ruler, Rowe is now measuring the space in the opening between Danielle's chest wall, end to end. "Now that we've spread her loose, look how her lung bubbles up. She's got plenty more room to breathe."

"It was four centimeters before we started the procedure, and now we've gone to nine centimeters," says Smith. The anesthesiologist estimates that Danielle's breathing has immediately been improved by 20 percent.

"What kind of life expectancy does this child have?" Joe Collela asks.

"This is the longest living survivor of Jeune's syndrome right here," Rowe replies. "We saw a lot of kids die until we tried this first operation with this girl. I'm not sure it was such a good idea, but we kind of got attached to her."

In addition to his immediate concern with Danielle, Rowe has become increasingly involved with the fate of a three-year-old Navajo Indian child from Farmington, New Mexico, Rollandrea (Rolly) Dodge, born with intractable diarrhea, which prevents the absorption of necessary nutrients. Although she could occasionally eat a snack by mouth, primary nutrition was supplied through TPN (total parenteral nutrition) intravenously, a safe procedure in the short run, which can in the long run—and in this case did eventually—lead to liver failure. Rolly was originally referred to Pittsburgh, the largest organ transplant center in the world, to be considered for a liver transplant, but Rowe and pioneer liver transplant surgeon Thomas E. Starzl were now beginning to believe that the only procedure that might save her was a highly experimental multivisceral (in this case, five-organ) transplant.

This multiorgan transplant had actually been attempted a few other times, first in 1983 by Starzl on a child whose insides had been destroyed in a swimming pool accident, and in one other case—both leading to almost immediate death. But in Pittsburgh in 1987, the procedure attempted by Starzl and his transplant team on three-year-old Tabatha Foster, a black child from Madisonville, Kentucky, with an ailment from birth similar to Rolly's, showed promise. On the negative side, Tabatha had not been able to eat solid food after the surgery and had also not recovered enough to leave the hospital. On the positive side, Tabby had lived seven months and had easily avoided the rejection problem (the body's natural immune system will invariably attempt to reject the organ implanted into it) plaguing many other organ transplant recipients.

To Thomas Starzl, who had pioneered liver transplant surgery in the 1960s and 1970s, losing the vast majority of his patients, Tabatha's surgery represented enough progress to try again. Rowe, on the other hand, was not necessarily in agreement, and his reasons were personal as well as scientific. He was not certain that enough progress had been made in analyzing the data supplied by Tabatha to justify another procedure. In addition, and perhaps in some respects more important, he had become inordinately attached to Tabby, who, like Danielle Burdette, possessed an incredible ability to endure agony while maintaining a cheerful and silent presence. "I'm not sure Tabatha is going to die," Rowe once told me. "But sometimes I think that I will die if she doesn't get better."

Now the ortho nurse has reappeared, carrying the threaded rods—with matching nuts and washers—that Rowe had previously selected. Rowe screws the nuts onto the rod to see how smoothly they will fit, but he doesn't like the look or feel of the washers, and he directs Smith, and Michelle Scaletta, a physician's assistant in the Department of Surgery who has come into the OR to observe, to make new washers out of epoxy. They immediately begin mixing and stirring a powdery substance with water on the back table of OR #7. "Like making biscuits with Grandma back home," Smith says.

"I want those washers nice and thin," says Rowe.

"We'll make 'em like Necco wafers," Smith says.

"These rods, or 'pins,'" Rowe tells me, "are usually used for broken bones in legs. No one as far as I know has ever used them for chests."

Although this procedure has never before been attempted, it is elegantly simple and creative. Marc Rowe is trying to provide Danielle's lungs with more space to expand, but also, because the sternum or chest wall has not grown to accommodate and protect the lungs, now released from two years of confinement, he is attempting to construct a new chest wall the way the frame of a plaster-of-paris sculpture might be fashioned. The rods that Rowe has carefully selected will serve as surrogate bones.

A brief lull occurs in the OR as Rowe and Teich wait, hands cupped together, for the homemade washers to harden. When they are finally ready for use, Rowe picks them up in his gloved hand, stares at them carefully. "Good job," he says. "But I think I'm going to use the washers that actually match the nuts. These others," he says, "seem a little awkward."

"Well, we tried," said Smith.

"I appreciate it," said Rowe. "But I gotta do . . ."

". . . what I gotta do," says Suzanne.

Teich, aided by Rowe, inserts the blunt end of the metal rod into a small, ordinary-looking hand drill. There is a sharp point at the other end of the rod, and he pushes that point into Danielle's chest wall. He screws a nut and washer all the way down the rod to the side of the chest that has already been punctured, then tightens the nut against the chest by turning the drill rapidly. He next punctures the other side of the chest wall, screwing in another nut and washer and tightening it similarly with the hand drill, then gives each nut and washer combination an extra turn with a tiny hand wrench. The surgeons repeat the process twice, so that within twenty minutes, three metal rods, from four inches to six inches long, form the superstructure of Danielle Burdette's new and expanded chest.

The tools and equipment with which Rowe is working have oddly skewed the atmosphere, almost as if we are in a workshop in the back of a gasoline station rather than an operating theater. To further enhance the illusion, Nancy pulls a large thick hydraulic hose from the ceiling and attaches it to an electric grinder, called a "burr" (the Ortho nurse could not procure an appropriate file from Maintenance). Rowe triggers the tool, and with tiny metal flecks flying everywhere, glinting like golden lint under the bright spotlights, quickly eliminates the threading from each of the three rods, flattening the tops.

Now Rowe is wielding an industrial-sized wire cutter. "Watch your eyes; turn away," he says, as he clips off the ends of each of the rods. One after another, six bits of metal rod shoot across the operating room. He reactivates the burr and smoothes down the ragged ends of the rods so that they are flush against each nut and washer. Nancy hands him a plastic squeeze bottle filled with warm saline solution, and he washes Danielle's chest carefully until he is certain that all of the metal shavings have been eliminated. "Let's keep irrigating the chest like hell," Rowe says. He stops for a second to put his finger on a cute little jumping ball adjacent to the lungs, which we all ponder with momentary awe: this is Danielle's fist of life—her heart.

Periodically, Rowe will ask the anesthesiologist to exaggerate a breath by pumping more air and slowing the breathing, so that he can watch the lungs fill and empty. Although Rowe seems satisfied, Smith is troubled by the fact that the lungs press up against the rods. "That wouldn't happen if the rods were curved."

Rowe responds by attempting to bend the rods with his hands, but he cannot get a good enough grip to do the job. "Bring me the benders," he says.

"Do you think twenty percent improvement in breathing is satisfactory?" Smith asks. Looking back in Danielle's chart, Smith has discovered that Danielle's pulmonary function had slipped by 20 percent over the past two years. "So we're just breaking even," he says. Smith suggests that Rowe repeat his first procedure, expanding Danielle's breathing potential by removing a rib on both sides of the sternum. But Rowe is clearly reluctant to entertain more surgery and changes the subject. "How the hell do you use these benders?"

Suzanne explains the general principle, and after a shaky try or two, he quickly and efficiently curves each rod into a kind of semicircle.

"Now what do you think, Sam boy?" he says to Smith.

"Now I really like that," Smith replies.

"But now I don't," says Teich. "This whole thing makes me nervous. What happens if the rods get flipped around? Then they could dig so deeply into her lungs that the lungs could be punctured."

"Well," says Rowe, "maybe we'll make a support to fuse all three of the rods together: a brace." He asks Michelle if there is any of that epoxy stuff remaining.

Up to this point, the entire surgical team has been moving at a relaxed pace, but now they all seem to have simultaneously caught a second wind, for the activity quickly becomes more rapid, while the collective mood in the OR seems somewhat more intense. Danielle is not in danger, but these added adjustments to Rowe's creation have extended the procedure longer than expected, enhancing the general suspense and anxiety. Michelle spreads the epoxy, which is hardening quickly, on a plastic sheet. She uses a tongue depressor to cut three long strips, and hands them all over to Rowe.

"This is pretty damn sticky."

"Well, that's so you can mold it," says Smith.

"Just like a good surgical resident," says Rowe. "Sticky but easily moldable."

Kneeling over Danielle, he makes a thick band, perhaps an inch wide and an eighth of an inch thick, molding it around the rods, like clay. Now comes the Gortex soft-tissue patch to form a lining between the frame that has just been fashioned and the sternum and lung. Then Rowe and Teich quickly sew the Gortex directly into the sternum. Next, Teich pokes a hole into Danielle's abdomen and inserts a clear plastic drainage tube, primarily for excess bleeding. When the surgeons are certain that the wound is dry, the tube will be removed.

"Will this be her last operation?" Collela asks.

"I'll probably do this again one more time in about five years," says Rowe. "After that, I think I'll retire."

Chapter 4

AT 3:15 P.M., exactly six hours
after first cut on Danielle Burdette in OR #7, Marc Rowe pads
down the hall toward the Intensive Care Unit, to which his patient
will soon be transferred. Although there is a large waiting room,
with a television, tables, and magazines, in which she can often be
found following some of her favorite afternoon soap operas, Rowe
discovers Debbie today in one of the small private rooms adjacent to
the main area. Chaplain Leslie Reimer, an Episcopal priest assigned
to Children's Hospital and Presbyterian-University Hospital by the
diocese to serve the organ transplant community, has been waiting
with Debbie through most of the day.

Reimer, the first and only chaplain whose congregation is exclusively organ transplant recipients, with Debbie and Danielle as a
rare exception, has undoubtedly witnessed more pain and suffering, more often, than anyone else in the hospital, surgeons and
nurses included. It is an unfortunate reality that the support of a
clergy person in a major medical center is sought almost exclusively
when danger is apparent or death is imminent. At Children's,
Reimer conducts the regular holiday services, as well as the monthly
memorial services. She sits in vigil with families when children are
dying and then supports the medical staff at the bedside for hours
and days after the death.

With deep circles under his eyes and a face gray with weariness,
Rowe slumps down onto a sofa along the wall and briefly discusses

the procedure with Debbie, joking about how the new chest he built will enhance Danielle's measurements. "Last time we did this, she wanted me to buy her a T-shirt. You know what she's going to ask me for now? A bra!"

Debbie is concerned with Danielle's pain. "Will she be paralyzed [sedated]?"

Rowe assures Debbie that Danielle will be comfortable. "The real problem is infection," he stresses, meaning any sort of tissue or viral problem, including pneumonia, to which Danielle is quite vulnerable. "If she gets infected, we will have to take everything out, all the materials, the foreign body I just put in. And if we have to do that, I will tell you right now, it'll really be terrible." Rowe does not need to mention the additional complications pertaining to the stent or Danielle's trachea—problems that have yet to be solved.

When we first walked into the waiting room, Debbie, who had been crying off and on through the day, seemed quite tense and fearful, but as Rowe continued explaining and joking, the strain reflected in her face began to ebb, and before the end of the ten-minute conversation she was nearly smiling.

Rowe had personally selected Debbie Burdette and Trish Cambron for me to meet and interview because they could most accurately and honestly provide me with the "opposite side" of the relationship between the surgeon and his patient. Rowe was fascinated by the subculture and the camaraderie that exist at Children's between the families of patients with chronic health problems, especially those mothers like Trish, Debbie, and Tabatha's mother, Sandy, who, fearing that the physicians would not permit the highly experimental multiorgan transplant for her daughter, had "gone public," inspiring the local black community to rally in her daughter's support. It was this threat of a public outcry, along with Sandy's steadfast and unwavering commitment to her daughter, that had tilted the scales in favor of proceeding with the surgery, despite the overwhelming odds against success.

Few dynamics are more convoluted than those emerging between a mother and her child's surgeon, who, on a very basic level, has never been forced to put much thought or energy into the art of conversation and communication. Surgery itself is difficult enough. With each procedure—dozens each week—another life has been placed in his hands. But the size, delicacy, and innocence of the child complicate and intensify the challenge. An hour, or many hours, later, emerging from this private and intimate world, surgeons are usually numb and exhausted, anxious to eat and sleep, to make contact with their families. Yet the families of the patients upon whom they have operated must be tended to, questions answered, courtesies observed. At a time when every ounce of strength and emotion have been drained from them, compassion and sensitivity are of paramount importance.

Even with surgery finally completed for the day, they cannot sleep or go home, for they must round (do their rounds); they must examine the patients operated on yesterday as well as those slated to go under the knife tomorrow, responding to questions, comments, and complaints from assorted family members. If any of these patients suffers from dangerous complications, the surgeon must respond by returning to the operating theater immediately. (That day, Rowe remained in the hospital, attending meetings and rounding on his patients, until 10 P.M., nonstop.) All the while, the families, especially the mothers, are hovering, insistent in their worry and their obsession.

Trish Cambron was not alone in her feeling of surprise and resentment toward Rowe's lack of courtesy, but Rowe's colleague at Children's, David Lloyd, who met Rowe at a conference in South Africa (Lloyd followed his father in practice in a small hospital in the outback), maintains that Rowe is not selective in his rudeness. "I learned long ago that if I'm sitting right here, and he walks past me and ignores me, it doesn't mean he's mad or doesn't like me. It just means he's thinking about something else. People take it very personally, however.

"He's also rather blunt and tends to tell people they're dumb when he thinks they're dumb. So it's very easy for people not to like him. What they don't appreciate is that underneath, he really cares about people liking him. You often find that people who have this aggressive, gruff exterior are actually quite sensitive underneath. Very shy. At a cocktail party, Marc—and I'm somewhat like that too—is disastrous. We'll stand in the corner and drink beer and not meet people, because we have this block about reaching out and shaking hands."

If surgeons are reluctant to get involved with a parent, it is not necessarily because they lack compassion and shun conversation, it is more the practical element of time. "The pediatrician can make rounds and see all his patients, and that's his job for the day," says Lloyd. "I make rounds and I see my patients and I still have to go operate—sometimes ten hours in the OR. I also have to do outpatient clinics, just like the pediatrician. I don't have time to sit down and talk. I like to see the patient, make a diagnosis, operate, fix him up, then go on and help somebody else."

These facts of a surgeon's life make a mother's existence very difficult. These women have been charged with the unending responsibility of protecting a child they have brought into this world, cared for, sat up with nights, and worried over, seeing to it that they're fed and kept clean and have what they need. Being a mother at a hospital, says Trish Cambron, means being a soldier, fighting against all dangers and distractions, including poverty and sickness and the stubborn idiosyncrasies of exhausted surgeons.

After a while, she says, nothing in the world seems very important to you other than the child you are sworn to protect. You lose your connection to home, and at some point you lose your connection to your friends, the other members of your family, to your husband. You don't have a sexual relationship anymore. Your overwhelming concern is always the health of the child, and it so dominates your consciousness that you can't, you won't focus on anything else.

Although Marc Rowe feels that he is often in combat with these driven women, he understands and has learned how to live or coexist with their obsessions. Rowe says that many of the mothers with whom he deals are women who have cared for chronically ill children for long periods of time and to a large extent have become physicians to their own children. "I always tell them there can only be one doctor on the case. I'm willing to listen to every suggestion, but I'm the one who makes the decision. What I say to them is, 'You have to have faith in me. I don't care whether you like me or not. My only real job is to give your home a healthy child, and if I can do that, you're going to love me, even though you might hate my guts.'

"Sometimes I get very attached to parents. I feel as close to them as I do to my own family. But I don't let that sway me. I'll dump on them in a minute, because basically, I'm cold-blooded as hell about one thing—I'm trying to get their kid to live. That's why I have fights with pediatricians." He is referring to the fact that he has been urged to be more tactful and less aggressive with families of chronically ill children and their parents.

"Psychologic trauma and all that stuff is important, but it doesn't make a goddam difference if you're well adjusted and dead. Let's save a patient's life, and then we can get somebody to straighten out some of the hangups they get in the process. But if they're dead, it ain't going to make no never mind.

"The problem is—and this happens, honest to God it does—you begin to start changing the way you treat the child because of your attachment to the family. I don't want to do that, and I don't think it is good for the child. It's like my wife says: 'I don't want a pediatrician who massages me, I want somebody that takes damn good care of my kids.'" At the mention of his wife, his voice falters. A shadow flickers through his piercing brown eyes, and uncharacteristically, Rowe turns away for an instant.

In confirmation of Lloyd's observations that surgeons like Rowe lack an understanding of the norms of the real world, Rowe's wife of thirty-two years, Joyce, told me that her husband, as talented as he is in the operating arena, has no real conception of certain basic courtesies, such as casual salutations. "He doesn't realize that if you say good morning and smile that it means something to other people. It's important. In fact, he actually tried it out in the hospital for a while, greeting people, and one day he said to me, 'They smile and they say good morning back.' So surprised! He's often very distracted; he's a lot like the typical absentminded professor."

Whether it is actually absentmindedness or simple self-obsession, I have found surgeons, especially the most successful, such as Rowe and Thomas Starzl, to be some of the most detached human beings I have ever known. They are basically unaware of the clothes they wear, the lack of style and/or color coordination. They are often unaware of other aspects of personal hygiene, such as their two-day stubble, their sour breath. They are unaware of the simple basics of modern life, such as the need to carry money around the hospital (for lunch or dinner) or wear beepers like most other physicians, or wristwatches, or make the slightest pretense of following a schedule or meeting appointments. They are often unaware of other people's feelings. Rowe is less eccentric than Starzl, but admittedly triggered by mysterious forces he describes as "the little men in my head."

Joyce Rowe understood her husband's obsession with surgery from the beginning of their relationship. A friend who thought that a young unmarried nurse should come to know an up-and-coming single surgeon had arranged a meeting. On their first date, and on many dates thereafter, Rowe would drive by the emergency room of Boston City Hospital, and if the entrance looked crowded with cars, he would tell her, "Do you mind if we put this date off for another time? The ER looks busy tonight and I might get the opportunity to do some extra suturing."

As to how they have managed to live together over the years, Joyce Rowe says, with a look of capitulation and a sigh of acceptance, "I have a philosophy about doctors that fortunately agrees with his. That is, if you're going to be a doctor, then you should be a good one. I would like my doctor to be available to me when I need him. Therefore, I feel that way about Marc and his patients. Without my feeling that way, it would have been extremely difficult.

"And when you come right down to it," Joyce Rowe observes, "there's not a lot to get angry about with my husband. He doesn't have a drinking problem, he's not out running around with other women. I always know how to reach him, where he is—in the hospital. How can I be angry at a man who is out saving a child's life?

"I think the one adjective that I would use in describing our life, however, is 'lonely.' We've been married for thirty-two years, but out of that, I don't know how much I have actually seen him. I think he's been a very devoted husband and father. When things are impor- tant, he's always there—for me, for his children, and for his friends. It's still a lonely life, however, and I think I am more lonely now than ever before, since over the past year all of our children [four] have gone. So I'm much more aware of his absence now than when the house was full of kids." Joyce Rowe says that she knows that lately her husband is trying to make up for the past, that he is trying to spend more time with her and talk to her more when they are together. "But it's so hard for him. The man is so terribly distracted and committed."

With a quarter century of perspective to guide him, Marc Rowe once told me that he is not completely certain anymore that he has made the right choices. "I think the only regret I have, really have, in my life, is I should have treated my wife better over the years. I think I did reasonably well with the kids, but I would say of my own marriage, looking back, I think that's the one thing I have a lot of regrets about. I was very selfish."

"Do you treat her better now?"

Rowe shrugged. "I haven't been home for more than a couple of hours this whole week, and we are right now in the throes of getting a house appraisal, so that we can get a new mortgage.

"The house is in shitty shape, the faucets leak, and there's leaves all over the place, and she has to face an appraiser, and I haven't been home. I got home Saturday afternoon, I ran to the Salvation

Army to bring a bunch of junk in. Got home yesterday late, went to the dump before it closed, tried to fix the faucets, bathed the dogs, and did a few other things that she can't do.

"Periodically, I think about the time when our first daughter was very sick, and had a high fever, and she wanted me to take care of her, and my wife told her that I couldn't be at home because I was with a sick baby.

"And my daughter said, 'I'm a sick baby, too, Mommy.'

"That bugged my wife, it bugged her plenty.

"I kid the residents here by telling them that when they start this residency what they ought to do is have their testicles amputated, put them in the freezer, and then we'll reattach them sometime in the future."

As we sat in the cafeteria of Children's Hospital late that afternoon, Marc Rowe devouring a container of yogurt, then dipping the last of a large soft pretzel into a paper cup of yellow mustard, Rowe and I rambled through a gamut of subjects: his sense of guilt for not being in the hospital when Tabatha Foster died, his inability to understand Tom Starzl's own unique brand of obsession, the impending death from cancer of one of his colleagues (a man whom we both very much admired), his daughter's recent very nontraditional wedding at a rustic lodge in a nearby county park—but he actually had a special item on his agenda to discuss.

"Lately," said Rowe, "I think I have been thinking too much. I have been wondering, going over in my mind, some of the things I have done in my life, the sacrifices I have forced myself and my family to make. I have been asking myself questions I have always avoided asking before: How much of what I do is self-centered? Is it my own ego and my own image of myself and my own ambition to be somebody important that drives me so hard? What's selfish and what's idealistic? Where does one cross the line? How can a man go about unraveling the mysteries of life that energize, invigorate, and entrap us?"

Part II

The Pediatric Personality

Chapter 5

BRUCE ROSENTHAL, a soft-spoken, baby-faced pediatrician, was the preceptor that evening—the principal teacher, and one of five full-time attending or supervisory physicians who oversee all Emergency Room activity. Hours before the frantic pace of the night began, I found him sitting at the counter in the Physicians' Room, adjacent to the nurses' station, examining the early evening's ER activity sheets, humming along with a tape deck playing in the nurses' station. He had almost completed the first verse of a hearty rendition of "White Christmas" when second-year resident Laurie Penix, from Akron, Ohio, walked into the room and dropped into a chair opposite him.

In addition to the preceptor, the Emergency Room at full complement (evening shift) includes at least two second-year residents, one third-year resident, and two "interns," or first-year residents. Seventeen interns are accepted at Children's annually, through a complicated "matching" process involving 16,000 medical school graduates vying for slots in 4,500 programs across the United States. A little less than 10 percent of the 16,000 are seeking pediatric positions. Five nurses and a physician's assistant usually staff the Emergency Room, along with at least one rotating resident from an institution other than Children's. Some of these institutions have pediatric units, but few have units large enough to make the experience beneficial for the young doctor-in-training. In all the medical services combined, including surgery, approximately 135 residents will be working at Children's Hospital on any particular day.

In the Emergency Room, second-year residents shoulder the brunt of the activity, assuming responsibility for the critical-care rooms and the OBS (observation) beds, where the wheezers (asthmatics) are usually located, as well as a scattering of other patients. In 1988, the Children's Hospital Emergency Room handled more than a thousand outpatients a week.

"This is a five-year-old boy who fell on his way to school and landed on his face and head," Penix says. She is short and slightly heavy, with a tendency to talk too fast, a habit you quickly develop under the constant crush of twelve-hour days and seventy-hour weeks as a pediatric resident in a major medical center. "Before his fall, he complained of dizziness. After the fall, blurred vision. Initially, when he got home, he had blood coming from his mouth, nose, gums. He is somewhat sleepy, but his drums [eardrums] look normal. Everything normal."

Penix, who is younger by two years than most of her classmates because of the accelerated medical school program from which she graduated at Ohio University, stares down at her notes, scribbled on scrap paper, and doodles with her pen as she waits for Rosenthal's response. Halfway through her three-year Children's Hospital residency, she much prefers not to lean on her preceptor. But she admits that she is confused, really has no idea what to tell this anxious mother. Rosenthal, stocky, with rounded, soft features, asks a couple of general questions pertaining to patient history, then stands up and walks down the corridor toward Examination Room 5.

Upon entering, Rosenthal introduces himself to both mother and child and listens carefully, periodically nodding and asking more questions, as the mother once again recounts her son's symptoms. Usually, while conducting these interviews, Rosenthal will try to position himself at approximate eye level with parents and child. "But in this case," he later explained, "the kid was on the examination table, higher than Mom, so I sat up there with him."

"Does he get headaches?"

"I forgot to mention to the other doctor," said the mother, glancing up toward Penix, standing attentively behind Rosenthal, nodding occasionally and scribbling on a scrap of paper. "Yes, he has been getting headaches."

"Once a week? Once a month?"

"Maybe once a month."

Rosenthal examines the boy carefully, beginning with the eyes and working his way down. Finally, he places his forefinger on the little boy's thigh. "So what's this?"

"Toothpaste."

"What are you doing, brushing your leg?"

"Yeah, instead of my teeth."

Back in the Physicians' Room a few minutes later, Penix says: "The thing that impresses me is the fact that he landed on his face; he didn't even try to break his fall. How many kids would just allow themselves to fall on their face?" Penix's elbows are on her knees, and as she leans forward toward Rosenthal, she spreads her fingers and rotates her wrists so that the flat of her hands are parallel with the ceiling. "You know?" she says, pausing.

Rosenthal nods sympathetically. "One of the hardest things in medicine is to come to grips with uncertainty."

Penix and Rosenthal discuss the proper course of action—treat the wounds, get an X-ray; if no additional information becomes apparent, ask the mother to return with the child when the headaches actually occur. Later, over a cup of coffee, he tells me about the many unanswered questions in the world of medicine, and how young doctors must learn to deal with that ever-present reality.

"One of the things that people in training begin to learn as time passes, is that we are not going to be able to figure it all out. Oftentimes, the real challenge is how to present the idea to the parent that we don't always know what's going on. This is a big part of our job, and we must choose our words carefully. I don't like to say, 'I'm confused,' or, 'This is perplexing.' I want them to understand that it is not me who is confused. It is, rather, the situation that is not yet clear-cut.

"This is an aspect of the art of medicine—maintaining the parents' perception that you are a competent physician. One must learn to carry oneself professionally, acting in control, calm, and confident, not cocky and not deceptive, but able to leave them with the impression that they've come to the right place. I believe that there ought to be a little bit of the salesman in every doctor."

Physicians-in-training must also learn the proper way to ask questions, says Rosenthal. "You want to avoid yes and no answers, and you don't want to suggest an obvious answer. Sometimes I hear residents say, 'And you haven't had vomiting, headaches, back pain?' That drives me crazy! It's so easy to agree with a statement like that."

Rosenthal admits that despite his experience and position, there's a lot more about working in the ER and the handling of patients and families that he needs to learn. Usually, he says, the preceptor will not take patients unless it gets very busy. "When it gets backed up, I like to pick and choose what I take personally to vary my experience and patient contact." He prints ROSENTHAL on the patient-assignment chalkboard beside a child's name with VIRUS written beside it as the reason for the visit and walks into the examination room.

"Are you Danny or Daniel?"

"I'm Danny."

"Have you been out of school all week?"

"Yes," says the mother with aggravated emphasis. "He certainly has."

"Have you enjoyed that?"

"Yes," says Danny.

"But I haven't," says the mother.

"Have you ever had your throat tickled before?"

"He's going to take a culture," says the mother.

"That's right. I'm going to push your tongue down now," says Rosenthal, showing the child a flat wooden tongue depressor. "Now you pant like a puppy."

"No," says Danny, "I can't."

"Of course you can."

"No, I can't."

"Why not?"

"I don't know what to do."

Rosenthal puts the stick down and begins to explain what is going to happen and why the throat culture is necessary, that it will be "grown" in the laboratory in order to monitor for bacteria, but Danny turns away, becoming more upset. In an effort to help, Danny's mother attempts to intervene and provide direction, but Rosenthal waves her off. After many fruitless minutes of explaining, struggling, and cajoling, Rosenthal leaves the room. "We both need a break," he says.

Later, after Rosenthal returns to the examination room, the mother says, "Do it to me. I've had cultures done two times." Rosenthal shrugs and almost reluctantly complies. Seeing how it is done, Danny subsequently accepts the procedure with no complaint.

"It's interesting," Rosenthal later comments. "When a kid is afraid of the stethoscope, I'll usually say, 'Look. Watch me listen to your mom.' But I would have never asked her if I could do a throat culture. That's a bit intrusive. The mother saved the day."

Chapter 6

BRUCE ROSENTHAL'S difficulties with young Danny represent a primary difference—and challenge—inherent in the role of the pediatrician. In contrast to the more straightforward and clinical approach of the adult practitioner, pediatricians must cope with, among other things, the fact that their patients aren't necessarily going to communicate in a straightforward manner or express gratitude for the help the physician is providing. But the overwhelming majority of pediatricians believe that children, as patients, are a lot more forgiving than adults are when the procedure or examination being performed is uncomfortable or painful. Says Rosenthal's supervisor, Holly Davis, director of Emergency Services, "I think that kids have a real appreciation for what you do for them when it's all over."

According to Davis, it is essential for doctors and nurses always to remember both the psychological and physiological differences in children that make diagnosis and treatment considerably different from what they are for adults. "Children grow from very small to very large in the course of a childhood. Weight and vital signs change. Normal respiratory rate for a newborn is different from that of a one-year-old, which is different from that of a six-year-old, which is different from that of a fourteen-year-old. And the same is true of heart rates and blood pressures." Infants and children are more prone to hypothermia and dehydration. "Plus they're different behaviorally: infants and toddlers can't describe symptoms.

Pediatrics in some ways is much more like veterinary medicine until children are school age or older.

"Beginning around five or six months of age, infants tend to get stranger anxiety. If they see the parent's face, that's fine; they see somebody else's face, they start to cry. If they cry, it's tough to evaluate them, so when you are examining a baby six months to a year and a half, you don't want to look him in the eye. You want the parents to focus on the kid's face and distract him. Separation anxiety, which is somewhat different from stranger anxiety, follows when they are about a year old. Kids go into a panic when they are separated from Mom or Dad. So often, the better part of valor is to let their parents stay with them and participate when possible, whether it's transporting them in an ambulance or evaluating them in the ER." This philosophy in pediatrics—the idea of keeping parents together with their children—has evolved over the years and is in contrast to early practices, when parents were expected to relinquish their children to a pediatric institution for days, even weeks, with visiting privileges limited to Sunday afternoons, in order to keep the parents out of the way and to safeguard the child from infection.

The differences between child and adult, as well as infant and child, actually begin before birth, explains Shekhar Venkataramanin, a pediatrician in the Intensive Care Unit at Children's, with a special interest in the physiology of the newborn. "There is a critical transition phase, especially during the first week of the child's life, because the child's entire support system has been totally dependent on the support system of the mother. After the baby is born, the baby has to do everything by itself—breathe for itself, digest its food, make its own proteins in the body. So that first week especially, there are a lot of changes in the body, which are happening very rapidly, particularly in the lungs and heart. The circulation changes very quickly, and many of our critically ill patients that we have in the intensive care unit go in during that first week of life."

Children in all stages of development are more resilient and at the same time more vulnerable to disease than adults, says Venkataramanin. "They are fragile physically in the sense that it takes less of a problem to tip them over, especially if it's a very small child, but because they are so young and fresh and have not misused their body over the years, they have a much better chance of quick and total recovery."

It would not, however, be fair or accurate to say that adult institutions or community hospitals cannot care adequately for infants and children under certain circumstances. When the child's needs are relatively minor, and convenience dominates the decision-making process, a general hospital, staffed with competent pediatricians, is quite adequate. But when a child is faced with serious life-threatening conditions, children's hospitals are always preferable.

Even if the health problem is normally not life-threatening but may possibly lead to unforeseen complications, a pediatric institution may well be the appropriate selection. Carl Gartner, senior member of Gartner, Zitelli, Malatack, and Urbach, a group of pediatric generalists to whom community practitioners refer patients in need of hospitalization, recalls a number of horror stories when children who in most circumstances might have been adequately treated at an adult institution with a pediatric unit suddenly took a turn for the worse.

Gartner explains that the injection or inhalation of too much anesthesia during surgery or a minute inadequacy in hydration during an asthmatic attack, or even a momentary lack of attentiveness—all routinely minor concerns in the overall outcome of adult treatment—could and has meant death or disability to young people. One recent example concerns a patient with epiglottitis, an inflammation of the small structure near the root of the tongue which covers the entrance to the larynx when the individual swallows, thus preventing food and/or liquids from entering the airway. When the epiglottis is inflamed, it can cause sore throat, fever, croupy cough; it can interfere with breathing, and when untreated, lead to death. The diagnosis, Gartner explained, was made by a good pediatrician in a community approximately sixty miles from Pittsburgh, and although the intention was to transfer the child to Children's, the weather was unstable and a decision was made to care for the child through the night in the small pediatric unit of the community hospital.

Because the child was having breathing difficulties, the pediatrician and anesthesiologist intubated the child—placed a hollow tube into the trachea to protect the airway. This procedure in itself is extraordinarily more delicate and difficult in a child than in an adult. "Most tracheas in an adult are as wide as a quarter or fifty-cent piece," says Ryan Cook, director of the Department of Anesthesiology at Children's, "while in the average newborn infant, we're talking about the size of a small drinking straw." Cook defines the difference between an anesthesiologist trained in pediatrics and "my adult compatriots" as "the difference between a watchmaker and somebody who installs hubcaps on your car."

Meanwhile, the child was left in the unit to be cared for by the nurses, as was normal routine. "Everyone figured the baby would be fine," Gartner said. "But in the middle of the night the tube mysteriously plugged." These nurses were trained in pediatrics, said Gartner, but lacked the intense and varied experience of the critical-care nurse at most busy pediatric institutions. So it might have taken a little longer to recognize that the child was having breathing problems. In addition, the anesthesiologist who had intubated the child was on call but at home, "and there was no in-house ear, nose, and throat (ENT) surgeon, who might have been able to open the airway."

At Children's, with a surgical schedule of 10,000 anesthetic procedures a year performed by a staff of eighteen certified pediatric anesthesiologists, and at most other pediatric institutions, there are anesthesiologists and at least one ENT specialist in hospital and available twenty-four hours a day. In this situation, the proper personnel were eventually telephoned, and they rushed to the hospital, Gartner continued. "But by the time they got there, figured out what was going on, removed the plugged tube, and replaced it with another one, the child had died." Says Gartner, "I know that as a result of that episode, that particular hospital won't keep similar patients in-house overnight anymore." Gartner says that children, especially those who will remain in the hospital for an extended period, require "a total support package" offered only in children's hospitals, in addition to thorough and qualified care.

The support package to which Gartner refers is much more all-encompassing than most people would imagine. It not only includes surgeons, anesthesiologists, and other medical personnel specializing in pediatrics, but it begins with the building itself. "On a pediatric unit of an adult hospital," says Edwin K. (Ned) Zechman, Jr., president of Children's Hospital, "there might be Disney characters or Snoopy characters on the walls, but whenever the child has to go somewhere else in the hospital—anywhere from the cafeteria to physical therapy to radiology to the lab—the ambiance changes. The children's hospital, from front to back, floor to floor, has a unique pediatric persona."

Robert Sweeney, executive director of the National Association of Children's Hospitals and Related Institutions (NACHRI), which not only serves as a link between institutions but also represents the pediatric point of view to legislators and governmental administrators, primarily on a national level, explains that children's hospitals take care of 9 percent of the kids—400,000 of the 4.5 million kids who are hospitalized each year, not including births. "So when you come right down to it, considering all the attention and credit we receive—deservingly—we have an identity that is much larger than reality.

"Most of the one hundred thirty-three pediatric institutions across the U.S. are a part of a larger university medical center," says Sweeney. About forty of these institutions are free-standing and self-contained, and, like Children's in Pittsburgh, independent from the university with which they are affiliated. Some children's hospitals, although maintaining their independence, with their own board of directors and/or administrators, are actually a wing or floor of a larger physical complex. Many of these hospitals within a hospital were founded as free-standing institutions but later merged for practical and financial considerations.

"A classic example is the Floating Hospital at the New England Medical Center, which, in fact, was, back before the turn of the century, a ship used to haul the kids out into Boston Harbor so they could have the advantages of sunshine and fresh air—kids from the tenements of Boston. Then it got beached and was folded into the larger complex of the New England Medical Center. But it's still called the Floating Hospital in the curious way Boston does a lot of things. And there's still also a so-called Floating Hospital in New York—St. John's—really a diagnostic and ambulatory-care facility, which putts around New York harbor."

Zechman and Sweeney, as well as the vast majority of pediatricians, believe that children treated at an adult hospital, sometimes even for minor illnesses, will also be at a significant political disadvantage. Pediatrics is only one of many departments and programs vying for power, money, and influence within an adult health-care facility. Resources—equipment, supplies, research, and personnel—must be stretched in many conceivable directions.

Pediatrics specifically and child care generally have, historically, lagged far behind adult concerns. The very concept of childhood, down through the ages, has been generally ignored. In his writings, Philippe Aries, a prominent French cultural historian, notes that in medieval art up through the twelfth century, children were portrayed as little men and women, with complete adult characteristics and dimensions—writ small.

But today, within the confines of a children's hospital, the world is reshaped and the boundaries are redefined so that the child is the first-class citizen. Because many children treated at a children's hospital have fairly severe illnesses, their stay in the hospital tends to be longer and their diagnostic and therapeutic regimens much more complex. The children's hospital allows for these differences by providing more space per patient. Studies have shown that general hospitals range from 1,000 to 1,500 square feet per bed, whereas children's hospitals range from 2,000 to 3,000 square feet per bed and higher.

The trend in accommodations in children's hospitals today, reports Michael Tyne, a planner in the health-care field and president of Karlsberger Associates, a Columbus, Ohio, firm specializing in the design of pediatric institutions, is toward rooms "designed as virtual intensive-care units—private rooms that enhance monitoring, that enhance a team response to a patient medical problem, that enhance the provision of space for equipment, supplies, portable X-ray machines. The objective is to separate children with widely different disease categories, to provide privacy between patients of different ages, different sexes, different levels of intensity.

"We find that it's just not satisfactory to have a child who is near the point of being discharged from the hospital suddenly having thrust upon him a roommate coming out of surgery and in critically serious condition. We want to separate these kids, not provide them with the additional trauma of having to watch another child in the same room in acute distress, often reminiscent of the distress they have lived through." Tyne says that almost all children's hospitals are converting to an all-private environment, a fact that Ned Zechman confirms as an objective for his institution, not only for the overall comfort of patient and family but also for the benefit of the hospital itself.

"The reason I like a hospital that is all private rooms is because it gives you a great deal of flexibility in placing patients," says Zechman. "Right now, with two hundred ten beds at Children's, I can be filled at one hundred ninety patients, because of the wrong patient coming in. In an adult hospital, you can put a twenty-one-year-old and an eighty-eight-year-old in the same room, but in a children's hospital, I can't put a four-year-old and a fourteen-year-old in the same room, or a baby and a teenager. So that's why we want to convert to all private facilities." At 210 beds, Children's is approximately the twelfth largest pediatric institution in the United States, but it is also an international institution, its centers of excellence, such as organ transplantation, attracting patients from throughout the world.

Says Tyne: "The other thing that separates pediatric from adult facilities is the need to provide overnight accommodations for parents. We'll either provide a sofa that will convert to a bed, or some kind of recliner chair that is comfortable for the parent to sleep in." Children's of Pittsburgh also provides sleeping rooms for parents of children in the Intensive Care Unit; a more comfortable family atmosphere is available at the Ronald McDonald House, located ten minutes by automobile from the hospital.

"There's another problem in the children's hospital environment that relates to space," says Tyne. "A children's hospital has to have a variety of cribs, of youth beds, of full-size beds, bassinets, huge quantities of linen, gowns for patients of all sizes, from infants to very large teenagers. In addition, when a child is admitted to a hospital, you also have the parents, often grandparents, and siblings in attendance much of the time. That's more space and furniture." Even for the outpatient clinics, says Tyne, adults will often come by themselves for examinations and checkups, but for children, multiple seats must be available for the people accompanying them.

Because they are so specialized and because they serve a population whose behavior is so unpredictable, children's hospitals tend to be less efficient and subsequently more expensive than adult general hospitals. "You can take an adult patient into radiology and be reasonably certain that the patient will lie flat on the table," says Tyne. "When you tell them to take a deep breath and hold it, they will do so. But an infant, a toddler, will often move at the moment that the X-ray is taken; you end up with a blurred film; the film has to be retaken. When the laboratory technician or the phlebotomist goes into a patient room to get a blood specimen, the child is anxious, often screaming and crying. These are problems that mean generally lower productivity ratios. Hospital staff have to spend a lot of time calming the child, reassuring the child."

Another reason that children's hospitals might cost more has to do with their clientele. Because many families cannot afford a private community pediatrician, the children's hospital has become the family pediatrician to the urban poor. "We take care of their runny noses, and their earaches, and their tonsillectomies, as well as their more complicated ailments," observes Zechman. This responsibility also drains the institution of its assets. "About twenty-eight percent of the kids seen in children's hospitals nationally are covered by Medicaid, which pays seventy-six percent of the cost of their care—not the charges, but the cost. Cost is typically about eighty percent of charges." Ned Zechman says that Children's Hospital loses about $5 million on outpatient Medicaid patients annually.

Chapter 7

SPACE, furniture, supplies, equipment, and interior design and decoration represent only a small part of how and why children's hospitals differ from adult institutions: the primary component is the people and their special orientation to children. Each of the men and women in the hospital seems to possess a soft and pleasant style and manner—what some psychologists and people in the health-care field call "the pediatric personality." It arises from an affinity for children—or, conversely, an aversion to the destruction adults can wreak upon themselves.

In internal medicine, as well as surgery, the majority of one's practice is centered on patients who are sick or ill because of diseases of abuse—dietary or chemical—while a child's disease is usually devoid of societal baggage. Pediatrics presents for the practitioner an opportunity to start with a patient at the beginning rather than the end of life, to attempt to nurture and preserve what God and nature have so generously and miraculously provided. Children can restore your faith in medicine and in the world at large; they will make you smile, and they will keep you unpretentious. Gartner says, "It is difficult to be very stuffy if you're examining a small child who urinates on your tie."

"I often get myself in trouble because I describe pediatricians as 'warm and cuddly,' " says Robert Sweeney of NACHRI. "But there is that friendly aspect to them. And they know that in order to be effective, they must treat the whole family, not just the child. Frequently you hear surgeons described as brilliant: 'Brilliant surgeon—in spite of his personality.' But young families are attracted to a pediatrician on the basis of his aura, and then after that attraction, I think parents make some judgment about his professional skills."

As one might imagine in an atmosphere such as a children's hospital, surgical personalities and pediatric personalities will often clash. Surgeons usually wear the symbolic white hats. Surgeons, especially in the areas of pediatric trauma and organ transplantation, will, by necessity, act instinctively and spontaneously. They are action-oriented, not the type to answer the questions of both parent and child to soothe their fears and assuage their curiosity. "Save lives first," one Pittsburgh surgeon scolded a young resident who had stopped to talk to a family, "answer questions later."

Surgeons will also often ridicule their pediatric colleagues. "A pediatrician," a prominent Pittsburgh cardiac surgeon once commented, "is a doctor whose personality reflects the emotional development and maturity of his patients."

In some respects, this surgeon's ungracious comment rings with a certain truth: A good pediatrician or pediatric nurse, many of whom like to wear tiny stuffed animals on their stethoscopes and smile stickers on their identification badges, must be willing to crawl across an examination room floor in pursuit of a rolling ball, play jacks, or talk gobbledygook in order to gain the trust of the tiny patients they must diagnose and treat. But to most pediatricians, including many surgeons, this is a pleasurable bonus of the profession. "I love the idea that I can sit down with my patients and play with them sometimes," says pediatric nephrologist Ellis Avner. "I enjoy the idea that I can laugh around the hospital without being thought of as being strange, as in many adult institutions.

"I also think you'll find most of the people who go into pediatrics are much more concerned with issues of interpersonal relationship, of family, of future, of patient potential, and are willing to deal with some of the most difficult situations in health care to accomplish that. There is nothing," says Avner, "more tragic than dealing with a dying child. Nothing in the world. When certain colleagues criticize us, make fun, I always think about how they would face the realities of a high-acuity pediatric institution on a regular basis. It takes a special and insightful person—a real human being—to deal with children and their tragedies day after day."

Working at One Children's Place can be exceedingly pleasant, according to the Reverend Leslie Reimer, the Episcopal priest who ministers to the organ-transplant community at Children's—or it can be devastating. "The pediatric personality, by necessity, is a funny combination of never having grown up, yet being extraordinarily mature."

In the physicians' area of the Emergency Room, there are simultaneous conversations everywhere: between medical students and residents at the X-ray screen, between the preceptor and other residents, between residents and nurses. In a tiny, crowded lunchroom in the rear, residents and interns distractedly and quickly talk between bites.

"Molly, are you hanging in there?" Rosenthal asks second-year resident Molly O'Gorman of Buffalo, New York, who has just today returned from a two-week vacation. She is blond, short, and energetic, charging around the ER with her shoulders hunched forward, like a fullback.

"No, but I'm all right," she replies, rolling her eyes. "I just love my first day back in the ER."

"It was quiet all day until you got here. Nothing was happening until you arrived."

"I guess I'm a jinx," she replies.

Third-year resident Holly Frost comes in. "What are we doing about nipples? We don't have any nipples," she says, hurriedly opening and closing supply cupboard doors.

"I have no comment," says Rosenthal. "A person could crack a few jokes about that dilemma, but," he pauses, "it won't be me."

A nurse enters. "Who's in charge?"

"It depends on why you're asking," says Rosenthal.

"Well, we have a child here who at home is urinating on the floor, wiping feces all over the wall, then lighting it all with matches in the middle of the night after the mother goes to bed."

"In that case, the social worker is in charge," says Rosenthal.

Meanwhile, the phone is constantly ringing—parents at home and community pediatricians in practice seeking information and advice. O'Gorman talks to a pediatrician who asks a lot of questions about ER procedures. Finally, she slams down the phone. "He thinks we're sitting around here drinking coffee and eating," she complains. "He's watching television and crunching potato chips; he's got all the time in the world."

"When did you actually come on duty?"

"Just a few minutes ago," O'Gorman answers, "although it feels like I've been here since last September."

"I had somebody write a really nasty letter about me today," says Frost.

"So they found out about you finally," Rosenthal says.

"That's not funny," she says.

"Is it somebody you liked?" he asks.

"Somebody—parents—I liked and followed from the beginning of my residency, since their child was born. I was quite upset about it. I guess I won't see them anymore. But I wish they would have talked with me first."

Now, there's a discussion going on about cookie runs, an enjoyable but deadly serious tradition at Children's. When meetings occur in the hospital, department heads will frequently order coffee and dozens of fancy cookies from the Dietary Department. This happens throughout the day, and even into the early evening. Residents with spare moments will often lurk in corridors, searching for a recently evacuated meeting room, scarfing the leftovers before Dietary can arrive for cleanup and running down to the ER to share their booty.

Cookies traditionally are popular refreshments for residents at "morning report," at 9 A.M. each Monday through Friday, when the chief inpatient and outpatient residents, along with the residents working the wards, gather with the teaching doctors in the Department of Pediatrics to discuss the prior evening's activities and admissions. A resident is designated for a period of three weeks to provide cookies in the morning, as well as refreshments (food and beer) for Friday afternoon "fluid rounds," in the residents' lounge on the 8th Floor.

O'Gorman, who had left the room, now returns. "This kid I'm seeing now has been periodically constipated for six weeks, with bleeding around his stools."

Rosenthal wrinkles his brows and raises his forefinger in mock seriousness. "What does constipation mean?" He leans back in his chair, pompously folding his arms, nodding his head, and contemplating his student.

Monica, another resident who has been listening to the conversation, shakes her head, rolls her eyes. "I hate these philosophical discussions."

Chapter 8

AT 9:00 P.M., the Triage desk in the ER begins to back up—long lines of parents and children filling the chairs and spilling into the adjacent corridor. In Triage, a nurse will conduct a brief examination to determine whether the child should be seen by a physician—usually a resident—immediately or be sent with the parents to the waiting area adjacent to the registration desk, where they will be called in chronological order. Kids with headaches, stomachaches, burns, bumps, fractures, rashes, and ingestion are common. At Triage, the idea is to prioritize, to give children and parents the once-over.

Most children and especially parents will remember the name of their doctor, the color of his beard, the lint in his mustache, the crisp starch in his lab coat. They will hang on his every word, and later in the cafeteria over coffee, or in the car on the way home, deliberate on the nuances, the subtle meanings of his or her message. Never mind that the nurse took the vital signs and part of the history, that the nurse comforted the child and supported the parent during the examination, that the nurse explained what the doctor meant after the doctor left. Nurses are usually the anonymous faces and voices in a hospital setting—some resent it and others enjoy it. As nurse Cathy Stevens has discovered, however, anonymity, like it or not, is impossible while working Triage. During the busiest times, the nurse is the inevitable target of a parent's misdirected frustration.

"This happened just yesterday," said Stevens, "and it made me feel as if I never wanted to work a day in the ER again." She is twenty-five years old, very young-looking, smooth of skin and bursting with a blushing expectation of life that, as a nurse, at least so far, has never been achieved. "A father and a mother came in, new parents. They were afraid their baby was going to choke to death. So I took them into the [Triage] room and I said, 'Okay, tell me what's going on.' So they're telling me how this baby's losing its breath, a legitimate fear. 'Okay,' I said, 'I'll have the doctor check. You go back and sit down and somebody will see you as soon as possible.'

"There were about twenty people waiting, so I went out to the desk, started calling the next person. And as I'm standing there, the father runs out and he screams, 'My baby's choking, he's going to die, I need a doctor.' So I run in, of course. My blood pressure and my heart rate are off the wall, and I'm thinking, 'My God, this kid's arresting in my Triage Room.'

"But the baby was coughing on mucus like babies do, and I just said, 'Sir, your baby's fine, you'll see the doctor as soon as possible.' And he just started swearing and yelling, and telling me that I don't know what I'm talking about, and his baby is going to die, and you know, it was really a terrible feeling because he told me basically that I'm . . . I just thought he was going to hit me."

Never underestimate the effects of a child's illness on a loving, frightened parent. Even those parents who would, under normal circumstances, be staunch allies will often fall apart under the slightest strain. "I had one mother who was a nurse administrator from some other hospital, and her little girl fell on one of her father's tools. Just had a little cut. But the father started pacing. And then he started looking at me, glaring at me, and I knew what was coming. So I went over and I said, 'Is there a problem?'

"And he said, 'Is there a problem? Is there a problem?' And he started screaming, and then she, this nurse, started screaming at the same time. It makes me feel very upset that people do that. I want to say, 'I'm trying to help you. Why are you being so rotten?' "

Stevens, a graduate of Duquesne University, in Pittsburgh, has worked her entire career—five years—at Children's Hospital, three years on the orthopedics floor and two years in the Emergency Department. "In Orthopedics, the physical activity was tremendous. We would lift casts, roll people over, pick them up, put them down. I was constantly exhausted. But this place is more emotionally straining. I have a lot of nightmares and hospital dreams—not frightening as much as frustrating. You wake up and think, 'I've slept six hours, and I feel like I just worked another shift!' "

For nurses—especially those who enjoy nonstructured environments—the Emergency Room is usually a good place to work, according to head nurse Maureen Cusack. "You don't come in at seven o'clock in the morning knowing that your assignment will be six patients, how old they are, and what's going to happen to them, as you would if you worked the floors. In the ER, maybe you'll be in the critical-care rooms one day, Triage the next, or maybe you'll 'float,' filling in where necessary." Flexibility is paramount, as is teamwork. You have to learn to work together, shift into third gear, and constantly prioritize to get through the day.

Although clinically affiliated with the University of Pittsburgh and directly adjacent to its large, sprawling urban campus, Children's Hospital is an independent institution located at the edge of the largest ghetto in the city—an area known as The Hill, from which Stephen Bochco is said to have modeled his popular television series *Hill Street Blues*. Many parents who cannot afford a regular pediatrician will bring their children here for routine treatment or checkup at any time of the day or night. When this occurs, as it does perhaps a thousand times each week, the Triage nurse will often send children to the Walk-In Clinic, open twelve hours a day, which is also under the direction of the Emergency Department.

"But each kid who comes to this hospital must see a Triage nurse first," Maureen Cusack explains. This has been a steadfast and unbreakable regulation at Children's Hospital ever since a mother telephoned to report that her two-year-old son had fallen off the living room sofa. "She took him to another hospital, and they checked him, and X-rayed his skull, and said that he was fine, sent him home."

But then the mother phoned Children's—one of a hundred fifty "nurse calls" or "doctor [resident] calls" received in the ER each day—and was worried because her child hadn't urinated for a long time. "She was instructed by one of our nurses to push fluids—give him lots to drink—and if he didn't pee by six o'clock to come into the Walk-In Clinic. And that's exactly what she did. She came into the Walk-In Clinic at six, carrying the baby all bundled up. They were a little bit busy over there, not real busy, but she waited a short period of time, and when she was called into the room, the baby was dead."

A subsequent investigation confirmed the mother's story, at least to a certain extent. The child had indeed fallen off a couch, just as the mother had claimed. "But what she didn't tell us was that when they came back from the hospital, she [the mother] had beaten him. And he died in her arms in our Walk-In Clinic of a head injury. Now if the Triage nurse had looked at that baby the moment they walked in, that death might not have happened."

Just as Cusack had finished her explanation, an infant girl was rolled into the ER on a stretcher.

"I don't like kid calls," says the ambulance driver, whose name, lettered on his jacket, is Whammie. "You got a baby with seizures— get me a medic." Because EMTs (emergency medical technicians) receive only minimal pediatric training, they are often resistant to transporting children. This is the primary reason that Children's Hospital has its own specially trained pediatric transport team, who retrieve critically ill children from other hospitals.

The mother of the baby on the stretcher, a tiny woman with unkempt hair and battered running shoes, paused momentarily at the Triage desk to sign in. The ER sheet requires only the patient's name and age and a brief statement—just a few words—describing the problem. As the ER sheet is being filled out, the receptionist puts the child's name on a plastic identification bracelet and wraps it around her small wrist.

"Follow me," says Triage nurse Marianne Bove, who, as tonight's "floating" nurse, has relieved Stevens for supper. Bove glances first at the ER sheet and then at the families waiting in the line of chairs, who are observing the arrival of the infant with curious passivity. She lifts the baby out of the stretcher and carries her into Triage Room 1, smiling. "She's a pretty little thing," says Bove. "I've seen her before."

"She's always here," says the mother. "I need a pediatrician with office hours seven days and nights a week."

"Any history of seizure?"

"No, but I'm an epileptic, so I know what seizures are."

"How old is she?"

"About twenty minutes."

Bove, thirty-two, a four-year veteran of the ER, pauses and raises her eyebrow at the mother's answer but refrains from responding. Then she places the IVAC, the electronic thermometer, under the infant's armpit. "Can you make it beep?" she says, referring to the high-pitched sound emitted by the IVAC when body temperature is recorded.

The conversation finally plays back in the mother's ear—and she suddenly laughs. "Oh, I mean she's two years old, but this happened about twenty minutes ago, maybe half an hour. She was sitting on my father's lap. Her temperature was 105.4."

The IVAC sounds; Bove peers at the numbers. "It's not that high anymore."

"I'm an epileptic, so I'm terrified of seizures," the mother says. "My other child, a boy, he had a seizure a while back and got delirious, staggering around. It was awful."

"Your little girl is fine," Bove says softly, after a couple of minutes. "But I'm going to send you in to see one of our doctors."

Each time Bove completes an examination, she will send her patients either to the Walk-In Clinic or to the registration and waiting area for the ER, which is her choice in this particular case. "You go down the corridor to the pink panther"—a stuffed animal, four feet tall—"and turn left." Here a clerk will gather necessary financial information and punch out a blue plastic charge card, which will record each expenditure for later billing. Bove escorts the woman and child part of the way down the hall. Then she returns to the Triage desk, to scan the ER sheets and call the next patient.

The ER sheets provide an interesting insight into the kinds of medical and social problems with which the staff is regularly confronted.

"Complaining of side pain—103 temp"
"Hit his head in a car reck"
"Worsen since being here yesterday"
"Vaginal discharge—wart on finger"
"Stomache pains"
"Possible molesting"
"Hit head on wheelbarrow while sledding"
"Hirt arm"
"Fussie"
"Fever—sore neck—running nose"
"Appendicitis."
"Cut finger yesterday"
"Bad cold"
"I think he's sick!"

Chapter 9

THE wastebasket in the Physicians' Room in the ER is like an hourglass, measuring the shifts. By 10 P.M., the halfway point for those interns and residents who have started at 5 P.M., the basket is full, and by midnight—an hour before they can possibly begin dreaming about home, their warm beds, and their waiting spouses—it is overflowing with unused forms, candy wrappers, plastic containers, and unwieldy boxes from the fast-food places and pizza shops that ring the University of Pittsburgh campus.

Laurie Penix has dedicated an hour to patients in the OBS (Observation) Room, a wardlike area with six beds primarily for wheezers, who will be treated similarly with intravenous fluids— asthmatic episodes are often caused by dehydration—and an aerosol vapor to clear nasal and bronchial passageways. Ten percent of all short-stay medical admissions, in addition to another five hundred visits to the ER at Children's Hospital, are for children suffering from asthma, which can be triggered by allergens, air pollutants, cold air, exercise, and emotions, and occasionally by drugs. Asthma is not a trivial problem: approximately five thousand adults and children in the United States die annually from this disease. Especially during the cold-weather months, wheezers dominate the ER area, along with children suffering from middle-ear infection (otitis media), which will infect 85 percent of the nation's children at least once, at an annual expenditure for care and medication of more than $1 billion.

Evidence of otitis media has been traced by historians back to 1900 B.C. It can cause hearing loss and learning disabilities and can be life-threatening when permitted to go untreated for a few weeks or longer, according to Charles D. Bluestone, director of the Otitis Media Research Center at Children's Hospital, the largest center for treatment and research into middle-ear disease in the United States. Over the years, the center has "tried to evaluate the safety and efficacy of existing time-honored but previously unproven treatments for otitis media, such as tonsillectomy and adenoidectomy," says Bluestone. Chances are, the majority of the parents and perhaps the grandparents waiting in the ER at this particular moment have, as a rite of childhood, undergone one or both of these two procedures.

Bluestone and his colleague Jack L. Paradise, MD, medical director of the Ambulatory Care Center, have been instrumental in research that has significantly changed the pattern of thinking regarding treatment for middle-ear disease. In the past, there were two primary reasons for tonsillectomies: sore throat and enlargement of the tonsils. Infrequently, tonsils can become so swollen that they interfere with breathing or swallowing. Size was also offered as a reason for adenoidectomy. Says Paradise, "It was a presumption that ... they [the adenoids] probably had something to do with middle-ear disease. More often than not, the two operations were done together. . . . It was sort of, 'While you're at it, get both.' Years ago, tonsils and adenoids were blamed for many childhood societal ills, such as poor school performance and bed wetting."

In a wide-ranging series of clinical trials beginning in 1970, continuing through the present, and involving more than three thousand children, Paradise and Bluestone have demonstrated to the pediatric world that tonsillectomies can be "reasonable treatment for children who are severely affected with recurrent throat infection." Adenoidectomy did help some patients with recurrent otitis media, but not to as great a degree as tonsillectomy had for those with throat infection. Since Paradise launched his research and published his findings, he says, "tonsil and adenoid operations have declined drastically—from more than one million in 1970 to slightly under two hundred thousand in 1986."

Now O'Gorman replaces Penix in the OBS Room for the next few hours. Penix is called to one of the examination rooms to see a three-year-old named Kerri with stomach pains and frequent vomiting who has not stopped screaming since her temperature and brief history were taken in Triage more than an hour ago.

Penix carefully quizzes the mother about the color and consistency of the child's vomit and stools over the past three weeks, since the stomach pains began. In the course of the conversation, she learns that Kerri has been passing a lot of gas, that she hasn't been eating well, and that she's had a sore throat but not a runny nose. With the mother sitting on the examination table answering Penix's questions and the father pacing nervously in the background, the child has settled down. But the moment Penix reaches toward her belly, Kerri begins to thrash and bellow.

At first, Penix tries to talk and conduct an examination simultaneously: "Kerri, Kerri, do I have a red nose, Kerri? Look at my nail polish. Isn't that a crazy color, Kerri?" Eventually, the mother leans in to hold her daughter down, while Penix momentarily bypasses the belly and shines a light into the little girl's throat. "Real red throat. Now can I take a look in your ear and see if there's a bunny rabbit there? Or maybe a frog? Usually I say frogs to boys and bunny rabbits to girls. But maybe you're a frog kind of person. Would you like to look in my ear first?" Kerri momentarily calms down, but her struggle escalates even more when Penix slowly reaches for the belly. "I need to hear if your belly is growling, Kerri. C'mon." The battle of wills—adult against child—continues without relief for fifteen minutes, until Penix turns toward the parents with a sigh.

"Her belly feels really soft, which is good, but her throat is quite red. She doesn't have a fever, and that goes against an appy—I mean, appendicitis. And the fact that she is passing gas is a good sign, although it may well indicate a bowel obstruction." As Penix continues to explain, outlining the possible problems and the many options for testing, the parents seem to relax. Tension gradually eases from the mother's face, while the father, who had not once stopped pacing, leans exhaustedly against the wall. The suspense isn't over, concern still exists, but there is relief in knowing that a doctor is now in control of the situation, and that the serious problem—appendicitis—has probably been eliminated.

Outside the room, Penix opens her mouth wide and exhales noisily, miming a loud scream. "A kid in pain, real pain, will look at you without really seeing you and cry kind of blindly, but this girl just looked me right in the eye and screamed bloody murder. I'm sure this child is being bothered by something, but I am also certain

63

it is not too serious. A couple of weeks ago, I had another little girl, about eighteen months, who looked me in the eye in a similar manner. I wasn't even touching her, but first she screamed. Then I just stood there and watched as she sucked in air—and spat right in my face." Penix shook her head and then burst out laughing. "God, my ears are ringing."

Perhaps because she is younger than most of the residents at Children's, Penix is also somewhat more talkative and more prone to reflect her emotions candidly. "I cry fairly easily. And some of my lowest moments, especially during my first year as an intern, when we worked such long hours, were when someone would say to me, 'Laurie, you look like you're not having a good day.' And that's all it took—and Laurie was crying. I don't feel it's wrong to cry, but I hate crying when I don't want to. I think it's unprofessional to be seen crying," she says.

"And you know that people are going to say, 'Typical woman, falling apart, and crying.' Which is true. I am very emotional, and I think it's because I am a woman. I think if I'd been raised as a boy, I would have been taught earlier how to control my emotions. That doesn't make me any less effective as a doctor, however."

But according to another pediatric resident, Arcangela Lattari, the fact that she is a woman has occasionally diminished her value in the eyes of a parent. She tells of a family to whom she devoted the entire night, diagnosing a rare blood disorder and explaining it in detail, with a textbook, to the mother and father. As the long night turned into the dawn and the child was safely attended to and Lattari was about to go home, the parents asked, "When will the doctor see our son?"

Conversely, in her lonely and difficult work, Chaplain Leslie Reimer, only the second woman in her diocese to become an Episcopal priest, has discovered many instances when being a woman was an invaluable asset. "Moms seem to be more open with us; they express what's really going on in their minds in a way they might not if I was a man." Under the right circumstances, men—both fathers of the patients and even the children's surgeons—are also sometimes willing to relinquish their tough façade around women, says Reimer.

She remembers one incident with liver transplant surgeon Thomas E. Starzl, who, according to some observers at Children's Hospital, is a cold and difficult man, obsessed with surgery, while seeming to be generally unaffected by the personal plight of patients and families. During one liver transplant procedure that consumed nearly twenty hours, Reimer remained with the parents, as she will often do, until they both drifted into a fitful few hours of sleep, and then, instead of going home herself, decided to put on some scrubs and go into the operating room to assess the progress of the surgery. As a special chaplain to the organ transplant community, as the significant spiritual and personal link between patient and surgical team, Reimer has unusually easy access to every crevice and corner of the medical center.

She had intended to stop into the OR for only a few minutes that late night, she recalls. "I kept thinking, 'It's time to go home and go to bed now. It's time to go home and go to bed.' I didn't go, and I didn't go, and finally it was almost morning, and the case was almost done.

"I was just about ready to walk out the door, when they got into some real big trouble. For a while, I thought they were going to be able to rescue the child, but they weren't. It was a real volatile situation, because nobody wanted to see this kid die; the entire surgical team knew him, because he had been in the hospital and suffering with liver disease for a very long time." But he did die, said Reimer, despite a heroic attempt to save him.

"After it was all over, Starzl just sat down by the operating table. The kid was still there, soon to be cleaned up so that the parents could see him for the last time. For ten minutes, Starzl just sat. There was really not much of anything else going on in the room. The kid was dead. Starzl just sat. He was so quiet; it was such a contrast. Just minutes before, he had been so angry and so frustrated and so loud, screaming and swearing as the child had slipped away. Now he was just very still and very quiet.

"I walked over behind him and just put my hands on his shoulders and stood there. I don't know whether he even realized anybody was there, but that was a rare moment," a moment, Reimer adds, that she was permitted to share probably because she was a chaplain and a woman both. A man, despite his spiritual calling, might not have been as welcome. "He actually said a few sentences about how hard it was to go through what they were going through in the OR. But it was difficult for him to speak. It was really sad how he squeezed those words out."

According to a recent report by the American Board of Pediatrics Foundation, 50 percent of all women medical school graduates choose pediatrics as a specialty, followed by obstetrics/gynecology and then by psychiatry. But women pretty much remain second-class citizens in medical schools and even in pediatrics, when measured in a number of different ways, including compensation. "There is some evidence to suggest," the foundation report stated, "that women pediatricians' salaries are disproportionately less than men's for the comparative number of hours worked per week," an injustice countered in a comment by one young male physician on staff in the Children's Hospital Intensive Care Unit. "In pediatrics, you find that there are a lot of female residents and interns who don't hold up their share. They just don't. And in pediatrics, it happens more than in any other specialty because there are more women in pediatrics than anywhere else."

The findings by the board and the physician's comment come as no surprise to Ann Thompson, who has been the director of the Intensive Care Unit. (Thompson's responsibilities include the Neonatal Intensive Care Unit [NICU] and the Respiratory Care Unit [RCU], as well as the ICU.) As a member of the "last class of ten percent women" (up until a decade ago, most medical schools arbitrarily limited enrollment of women to no more than 10 percent of each class), she is particularly vocal and honest about the problems and challenges of women in a male-dominated institution such as Children's Hospital.

She feels that in comparing the productivity of men and women in the world of medicine, it is important to focus on the orientation of women throughout history and their dual responsibilities of mother and doctor. "We all grew up with images of what it is to be an adult," says Thompson, who has been married since medical school to pediatrician Joel Frader, also on staff at Children's. They have an eight-year-old son. "For most women that means that in addition to work, if that is your choice, you are also a wife, and you're a mother. You're home for your kids. You provide milk and cookies at the end of the school day, and you're the social organizer for the family. No matter how involved I am in my work, that agenda is always close to the surface. So whenever I make a choice—I may be here past bedtime and not get to put in my time at home—it's always measured against what I was supposed to be as a mother, as a wife." Guilt is a built-in and unavoidable handicap.

"It's real hard for me to devote myself the way men devote themselves," says Heidi Feldman, director of the Children's Hospital Child Development Unit. "I go home, I take care of my kids, and I think that that impacts upon how effective I am. I think if I could work about sixty-five, seventy hours a week, I could be a first-rate doctor-academician. But I don't. I work more like fifty, fifty-five on the average. I think if I weren't a woman I'd be working harder. So that's a problem." An article published in the Spring 1985 issue of *Nursing Administration Quarterly,* based on previous literature, concludes that there is "a suicide rate for women physicians four times that of women over age twenty-five in the general population. It is also approximately twice the rate for divorced women over age seventy—that group of women exhibiting the highest known suicide rate."

Children's Hospital surgeon Suzanne Ildstad admits that from time-to-time "harassment" has posed a difficult problem for her. "One attending during my residency decided he was madly in love with me. He harassed me at my house; he harassed me at the hospital. He gave me expensive gifts. He just totally lost his perspective. It put me in a very difficult position, because I was just a resident. This was somebody with a lot of power and a lot of credibility. I didn't want to just totally offend this guy and make him angry. I tried in a very tactful way to just have him stay away from me and leave me alone. Eventually he got the message."

Ildstad's husband is a physician at another center in the East, and so for the time being he is commuting to Pittsburgh on weekends—difficult for him, as well as for Ildstad and her relationship with her children, who initially blamed her and her new position at Children's for her husband's frequent absences. "My daughter used to cry every time we took him to the airport, and she'd say that she hated me 'because you take Daddy to the airport and you help him leave.' That's been hard, but the kids are getting much more settled now that we've got a good routine down." She hopes that her husband will find a position in Pittsburgh soon.

Ildstad is new at Children's, but Thompson, Feldman, and most of the other women there know that prejudice against women, albeit subtle and perhaps unintentional, does exist—and Laurie Penix and Molly O'Gorman might be proof of it. Even though eighteen of the twenty-two pediatricians in their third and final year of residency at Children's in 1988 were women, the two honored positions of chief resident (outpatient and inpatient) were both awarded to men. In fact, over the past decade there have been only one chief inpatient and two chief outpatient residents who have been women.

On the other hand, and perhaps because of the difficult battles she has been forced to fight over the years, Ann Thompson admits to being much more severe with her women trainees than with the men. "I'm a very harsh judge when women screw up. If men want to make fools of themselves, fine. But the women are carrying all the other women on their shoulders, so they better be good." This responsibility, along with a vague feeling of inferiority because of the inequity of their positions, often leads to unnecessary discomfort and embarrassment. Thompson, like Laurie Penix, is especially sensitive to the effects of her spontaneous emotions—crying under pressure or because of remorse or sadness.

She remembers a situation that occurred while she was working on a fellowship in anesthesiology (she is a board-certified anesthesiologist) at Children's Hospital of Philadelphia, before coming to Pittsburgh, when halfway through a surgical procedure a male colleague began yelling at her because he felt that she wasn't paying enough attention to the patient. "There are a lot of accusations you can make of me, but that's not one of them. I was angry. I finished the case, and it went all right. Woke the kid up, and the child went back into the unit, and that was that.

"The next day he [the surgeon] came up to me—I was so mad at him—and said, 'You're mad about yesterday, aren't you?' I said I was, and I started telling him why I was mad. I was so angry that I started to cry. He was mystified; he didn't understand. He just stared at me, disbelievingly. But you see, some people don't know how to eat their anger, and so they—usually women—displace it with tears. But then, unfortunately, to many men, you become this little girl who can be patted on the back and made nice to. That's what often happens and I hate that. It makes me angry.

"You don't see very many men dissolving in tears when they're strung out. I'm sure they're feeling it, but their defenses are different. Earlier this year, one of the women interns momentarily fell apart in front of me and one of the other women on staff, and she apologizes to this day for it. But it didn't matter to either of us. The idea that one can lose control of oneself is somehow very disturbing to us all, I think. That was eight, nine, ten months ago; she's subsequently proven herself to be a first-rate doctor."

Thompson's honesty and directness in the way she confronts her feelings and emotions have been demonstrated repeatedly in her attachment to and involvement with young Debbie Burdette and her little daughter, Danielle. Of all the patients and all of the doctors in the entire hospital, there is perhaps no stronger bond than that between Debbie and Ann Thompson. Some magic occurred; something clicked immediately between the older—Thompson was thirty-six at the time they met—professional woman and the helpless young mother who had suddenly found herself in this bizarre atmosphere.

"Almost at my first sight of Debbie with her little baby four years ago, I felt as if my soul was in it, was with them both. I have never been able to relinquish that bond—not that I would ever want to, either, for they are my babies, both mother and daughter."

She remembers vividly one recent instance when Danielle's condition was particularly vulnerable. "I came into the unit that morning, and I saw her in her bed in a near coma, and suddenly, at that moment, I really thought she was going to die, and I really thought a piece of me would die with her. Debbie picked up my fear instantly and just started to shake. Her whole body was shaking, and I wanted so much just to hold her and say it was going to be all right. But I couldn't. I couldn't give strength and confidence to Debbie because I didn't have it within myself.

"My crying over Debbie and Danielle Burdette lasted only maybe thirty seconds, but sometime afterward I found myself wanting to go back to the nurse and the surgeon who were with me and apologize. Then I thought, 'What is wrong with you? You don't need to apologize to anybody. What's wrong with feeling rotten?' How else can you feel, what else are you supposed to feel, when bad things happen to such innocent young people?"

Chapter 10

ALTHOUGH the hierarchy at Children's Hospital and the University of Pittsburgh is controlled on all levels—medical, academic, and administrative—by men, the hospital and most other pediatric institutions across the United States would not even exist if not for the compassion and dedication of women.

The hospital was inspired by the son of a prominent Pittsburgh physician, Frank LeMoyne, whose family had been active in the Underground Railroad during the Civil War. Kirk LeMoyne, who was eleven and curious about his father's patients and problems, came to realize that there were a great many children in the Pittsburgh area less fortunate than he and resolved to help them. In 1883, Kirk and a few of his friends formed a "cot club," which sponsored a "baby show"—a beauty pageant for neighborhood babies—with the intention of raising sufficient funds to endow a bed for children at a nearby hospital. Kirk LeMoyne's gesture sparked similar events, and within a few weeks, not only was a bed endowed, but surplus funds remained. These funds became the seed of Children's Hospital of Pittsburgh. On March 19, 1887, a charter was granted, and a voluntary medical staff was enrolled among physicians in the community who had a special interest in children.

At that time, there were actually few, if any, doctors who specialized in pediatrics (or "pediatry" or "pedology," as it was called then), and the American Medical Association had only officially acknowledged pediatrics as a specialty a few years before. The first meeting of the American Society of Pediatrics did not take place until 1889, when only a few children's hospitals were in existence across the country—most notably Children's Hospital of Philadelphia, founded in 1855, and Boston Children's Hospital, founded in 1869. Until then, the only institutions providing health care for poor and destitute children were orphanages and almshouses. On June 5, 1890, the first patients were admitted to a newly purchased and remodeled house started by little Kirk LeMoyne's act of charity: Pittsburgh Hospital for Children.

The hospital grew quickly. By 1894, there were 298 visits to the outpatient clinics and 213 admissions annually. Many of the first patients were foundlings—babies left on doorsteps. "I remember one year I saw a patient named 'John Doe Number 37,' " one observer noted in a diary published at the turn of the century. "He was the 37th little John Doe that had been received that year."

In 1894, a brace shop for orthopedic patients and a milk and ice station were added in separate hospital wings. At that time, many infants and young children suffered from attacks of acute gastroenteritis (labeled "cholera infantum"), with vomiting, severe diarrhea, and rapid dehydration, sometimes leading to death. Research led to the practice of boiling milk and storing it in an icebox, which resulted in a rapid decline in the illness. A fresh-air pavilion was opened in 1912 for patients with tuberculosis, which was a common diagnosis, as were rickets, constipation, indigestion, and scurvy.

If by today's standards the medical world was somewhat primitive in 1900, then the science of treating and caring for children was in the darkest of ages. Throughout the seventeenth and eighteenth centuries and into the nineteenth, women—mothers, grandmothers, maiden aunts, wet nurses, midwives, and nannies—were responsible for the care and treatment of children. By the middle of the nineteenth century, male obstetricians, whose interest focused on the problems of labor and waned at the birth of the child, instituted midwife-training programs—for men. The less women did, the better the doctors seemed to like it.

Women were permitted to raise money, however, or to participate in other useful ways in charitably oriented pursuits. With the exception of Dr. LeMoyne and his son, most of the initial 139 chartered subscriptions to the hospital were contributed by women, as was the first substantial bequest ($10,000), by Miss Jane Holmes on the occasion of her death in 1890. In addition to money, a great many supplies and equipment were presented to the hospital. Children's Hospital records show that Mrs. Grace Morehead furnished an annual Christmas dinner and gifts from Santa Claus for every child in the hospital. The Needlework Guild of Pittsburgh kept the hospital supplied with bed linen and children's garments.

In 1890, Mrs. Frances S. King's kindergarten class donated $150 for the purchase of an instrument case, and a group of little girls, all under twelve years of age—Marian and Lucille Mellon of the famous banking family among them—conducted a garden fair and realized the sum of $125 for the purchase of a microscope. The records show that every year more and more cots were endowed by women of famous families. In 1908, Mrs. Andrew Carnegie donated $2,000 toward the endowment of a cot or bed in perpetuity, with an additional $3,000 going toward the construction of a new laundry.

The average cost per day per patient at Children's Hospital was $1.40, and the maintenance costs for all the free patients in the hospital in the year 1909 was $19,714.67. In 1916, the telephone charge was $301.17, ice cost $985.80, fuel for heat totaled $3,276.61, and the light bill was $771. (Today, one hundred years after its founding, Children's Hospital has a total operating revenue of $84,814,245. Of this amount, approximately $43 million is for employee salary and benefits, while $31 million is targeted for materials, supplies, and services.)

As the institution grew, many of the most prominent women in Pittsburgh "took to the streets" to raise money for Children's Hospital. The event was called "tag day," according to a story in a 1913 Pittsburgh newspaper: "If some kind woman ties a tag on your coat or arm and holds out her hand for an offering, don't be angry. She's not doing it for pleasure, but for the sake of the helpless little children, nearly all of them cripples, who are in the Children's Hospital. They need your aid." There was also a flower day, when women on the street sold roses. In 1937, Miss Emilie Renziehausen donated a $1 million trust to establish and maintain a memorial ward for the study and treatment of juvenile diabetes, today a center of excellence at Children's. Miss Renziehausen had cared for a diabetic brother for more than twenty years.

Ironically, women were so successful in raising money for Children's Hospital that men began to become more assertive, assuming control of powerful oversight positions—primarily as members of the Board of Trustees, a governing body which, during the first two decades of operation, was composed entirely of women. From that point on, men became more deeply involved, and according to Walter Rome, an administrator in the 1940s and 1950s, an unwritten rule evolved over the years, by which only ten of the thirty-member board could be women, a ratio basically followed to the present day.

At the turn of the century, women also volunteered for many services at the hospital, such as working with orthopedic patients, making patchwork quilts, and making picture scrapbooks. There was a women's service committee, and one of their first projects was to organize a library and take books to patients. Members of the committee assisted the doctors in clinics as secretaries. Dressed in their yellow uniforms, they learned to roll bandages, sharpen and sterilize needles, and help patients in the whirlpool baths. Many members worked in the schoolroom, "hearing" lessons and teaching handicrafts.

According to an official history of the Volunteer Service Department, prepared by Mrs. Edward W. Demmler in April 1969: "After World War II, there seemed to be a nationwide realization that in-hospital volunteers—later called 'Service' volunteers—could benefit hospitals. Not only could they help at the bedside of patients, but they could also be called upon for secretarial tasks, receptionist duties, escorting of patients, entertaining of children and central supply chores. The Women's Hospital Auxiliary was established as a national organization sponsored by the American Hospital Association in 1952. The cherry red smock was adopted as its banner. A 1952 article, entitled 'Salute to the Ladies in Pink,' published in Modern Hospital Magazine said: 'They are giving hospital patients a kindly service that money couldn't buy.' "

Today volunteers in their red smocks remain a familiar and an integral part of the hospital milieu. In an average month in 1988, on some 641 occasions of service, 243 volunteers performed assigned duties in some forty areas of Children's Hospital for a total of 2,553 hours of service.

The first administrators or superintendents (chief executive officers) at Children's Hospital were also women and primarily nurses—six strong figures who wielded great influence and power. The last woman to serve (in the 1920s and 1930s) was a nurse, Laurel Bell Wilson, who, according to Harold Luebs, Children's Hospital's tenth administrator (in the 1960s and 1970s), was a great elitist: "When Miss Wilson wanted the elevator she had a certain way of buzzing—which would signal the operator to get everybody else out of the elevator and come to her floor directly."

The elevator operator in the middle 1930s was named Emil, and he, as well as many of the hospital's employees during that period, was handicapped, said former Children's Hospital director of personnel Dorothy Wallace. "He was a very bright man, and he had a lot of influence at Children's Hospital because everybody went up and down in the elevators with him. When Children's Hospital wanted to start a pension plan, the employees were to be assessed three percent of their salary, and they didn't know whether they wanted to do it. Emil thought it was a good idea, so while on the elevator each day, he persuaded all the employees to vote for it, and that's how we got a pension plan—because of Emil."

Emil and Miss Wilson, as well as a number of other employees, lived at the hospital during that period—an essential aspect of their compensation—and they got free breakfast, lunch, and dinner. "When I started at the hospital in 1938," said Wallace, "I got $42 a month and three meals a day. When they gave me an extra part-time job in the purchasing office, they increased my salary to $75 a month and three meals. My first raise after a year was $2.50 a month." Before World War II, pediatric residents received $41.75 per month as salary, after the war years, $75 a month. Today, they receive about $30,000 annually.

Laurel Bell Wilson was the administrator in 1923 when the original building that housed the Pittsburgh Hospital for Children burned to the ground. No lives were lost, and as the dining room, kitchen, administrative offices, and hospital smoldered, Wilson secured places for her patients at other hospitals throughout the city and transported them with the help of volunteer taxi drivers.

After the 1923 fire, the hospital was also quickly repaired (within a week) and reopened for operation, while the community united to raise money for a new and modern structure. The president of the Carnegie Steel Company, Homer Williams, thought a new fireproof, eight-story building was needed. Plans were made for a Children's Hospital fund drive, and there were so many volunteer workers that it was necessary to launch the drive at two separate hotels. The Pittsburgh team members met in the William Penn ballroom, and the Allegheny County team members met at the same time in the Fort Pitt Hotel, communicating by telephones connected to loudspeakers. The new hospital was dedicated November 1, 1926, as the first clinical affiliate of the University of Pittsburgh School of Medicine. The building cost $1.5 million. In 1954, a second building, the DeSoto wing, was added. And in 1986 a third wing, which included a six-story tower for patients' rooms and a heliport large enough to service the entire medical center—the cost, $100 million.

Laurel Bell Wilson was also in command when the 1936 flood inundated many parts of the western Pennsylvania area. In a brief and never-completed document, she recorded some of her memories of the night the flood water paralyzed the entire hospital, most of the city, and a good portion of the state.

"It began to be rumored that the power was going to be shut off. But we said, 'They would not dare to shut off a hospital.' This could not be. However, we began assembling candles, and I sent a social worker with a car to hunt candles in the stores. Our electrician canvassed the nearby hardware stores for flashlights, batteries, and lanterns, and he reported that no lanterns were to be had. Members of the Board scoured the County stores, expecting to find lanterns hanging from rafters, but the storekeepers laughed at them, saying that they had not kept lanterns for years. And then, as dusk was falling, the lights began to flicker, and with words suspended on our lips—we realized 'the lights are gone—the power is off'—and the silence was almost terrifying. No radios, no streetcars grinding their way home with the day's workers, no elevators, no machinery operating, but worst of all—darkness in the city." Two more days passed without power to many areas of the hospital, but with Wilson's strong leadership, the hospital was kept intact.

Money for all three buildings, according to Gayle Tissue, executive vice president of corporate affairs, the highest-ranking woman in the current hospital hierarchy, was raised through "capital campaigns," defined as a concentrated effort to approach corporations, foundations, small businesses, and individuals in the Pittsburgh area, as well as doctors, board members, and personnel within the hospital, for long-range pledges of financial support in order to fund "the bricks and mortar" of the building.

Capital campaigns occur only infrequently during the life of an institution such as Children's—unlike the annual fund, for which board members and volunteers solicit money from donors on a yearly basis. Tissue and her small staff were responsible for raising $17 million for the capital campaign to fund the patient tower and nearly $1 million for the annual fund, which was initiated four years ago. Income from the annual fund is utilized primarily for new hospital initiatives, such as start-up money for the bone marrow transplantation program or the purchase of new equipment. A new capital campaign, a $22 million effort for research programs, will be launched in 1990 to correspond with the hospital's centennial celebration.

Tissue's assistant, Rosalyn Markovitz, explains that annual funds and capital campaigns are part and parcel of most health-care institutions, but after ten years of experience in fund-raising, she finds that pediatric institutions (because of the children) are a special vehicle for people to contribute in very personal ways, such as with "planned giving" programs. According to Markovitz, many people have written Children's Hospital into their wills or set up trust funds in which income from an estate is funneled to Children's on a long-term basis. Contributors can specify what they would like the money to be used for.

She tells of a former teacher in the Pittsburgh public school system whose only child died in the early 1950s from polio—too soon for the Salk vaccine, developed in Pittsburgh a few years after. "The teacher decided to leave a third of his estate, which was $1 million at the time of his death, for a named research fund in memory of his daughter." One woman educated twelve unrelated children with income from her estate—and then donated the principal to Children's.

Currently, Markovitz has been negotiating with Sotheby's in New York over auction terms for a painting by an early impressionist artist, William Merritt Chase, which was dedicated to Children's at the turn of the century by the wife of a prominent Pittsburgh industrialist, H. K. Porter. The painting, an interior scene of a summer house on Long Island, hung in the medical library for many years, and then was unceremoniously dumped into a nearby closet, not to be discovered until a little less than two years ago, when a secretary with a fondness for art urged Markovitz to seek an appraisal. Sotheby's estimates the worth of the painting at a quarter of a million dollars.

Throughout its first twenty-three years of operation, any child who came to Children's Hospital was treated for free, but as time went on, the hospital found that it was taking referrals of more and more sick children whose parents could afford to satisfy their health-care debts. A pay ward was established, but the practice of providing free care to needy children has remained an inviolable tradition. "Free," by the way, does not mean that *all* treatment for qualified patients is free. And the program is not open to everyone in the United States. Usually, the hospital bill will be significantly reduced to make treatment affordable for families in western Pennsylvania, eastern Ohio, and northern West Virginia.

The Pittsburgh Press Old Newsboys, an organization of former newspaper vendors from all walks of life, was founded in 1926 by Max Silverblatt, who at the time was the *Press*'s downtown sales director. Money for patients at Children's Hospital was first raised through a one-day sale of a souvenir edition of the *Press* at Christmastime, but over the years the fund drive continued to escalate. Today, not counting corporate contributions, research grants, private endowments, or any other hospital-originated fund-raising activities, the community, encouraged by the *Press* and KDKA radio and television (Group W), whose on-air personalities are actively involved in soliciting funds, contributes more than $2.5 million to the hospital's Free Care Fund.

No other hospital in the nation, general or pediatric, receives as much for any similar kind of fund. Most of the contributions are generated within one month—from Thanksgiving to Christmas—primarily by concerned private citizens and business owners, including the largest supermarkets in the city, a prominent appliance store, and many fast-food chains and restaurants. National and international corporations contribute equally, staging promotions that stimulate income, a share of which (perhaps 10 to 20 percent of the gross) is given to the hospital.

Markovitz calls this concept "cause-related marketing," a trend that is beginning to catch on in other parts of the country. Cause-related marketing provides the opportunity for a corporation or business to give back to a community that has supported them but at the same time receive some reward, such as an enhanced local image, for their efforts. Children's hospitals are especially suited to be such causes, and some pediatric institutions, including Boston Children's and Stanford Children's, have recently launched similar campaigns.

For the free-care fund-raising efforts in 1990, to correspond with the hospital's centennial celebration, one prominent Pittsburgh restaurateur has launched a $1,500-a-plate seven-course extravaganza, with each course cooked by a great chef, such as Paul Prudhomme, Larry Forgione, and Jean Louis Palladin.

Markovitz, whose official title is assistant vice president of development, rarely participates in the actual free-care fund-raising activities for the hospital. Her responsibility is to represent Children's Hospital to members of the community, large and small, who feel that they want to dedicate time and effort to the fund-raising experience. She serves "as a sounding board and to walk them through the steps they need to tackle to accomplish their fund-raising objectives."

This includes the most significant efforts, such as the KDKA telethon the Sunday before Christmas, which generates about 45 percent of the entire free-care package for the year. It also includes people like Albert Lexie, who has for more than ten years visited Children's Hospital once each week, moving from office to office to shine the shoes of hospital executives, contributing a portion of his tips to the hospital. Throughout the year, Lexie also distributes contribution cans to businesses in his hometown in the Pittsburgh suburbs and solicits Christmas contributions from organizations such as the Rotary, Kiwanis, and Elks. In 1988, his efforts resulted in $4,440 for free care.

In contrast to the women of the medical staff, Tissue and Markovitz both feel that a woman's tendency to exhibit her natural emotions—"tears, dreams, laughter"—is a great advantage in her work. Tissue, thirty-nine, is the prototypical corporate executive, always impeccably but conservatively dressed, physically fit, articulate, and well educated. Markovitz is perhaps fifteen years Tissue's senior and is much more casual, outgoing, and expressive. Markovitz insists that a key to her success in her work as a fund-raiser, which she did not begin until she was in her early forties, after raising a family and sending her children to college, is her continuing effort to learn why people dedicate their time and money to Children's Hospital—or to any organization or social cause. "Commitment doesn't come out of the air," she says. "There has to be an emotional reason behind it."

I was about to ask if *she* had an emotional reason for working so diligently for Children's Hospital, sometimes twelve or fourteen hours a day. Markovitz must have sensed my question, because even before I spoke her face flushed and her eyes welled with tears. She told me two of her five children had suffered from a genetic disease and had died at Children's Hospital before their condition, today called aerial sufatase deficiency, an amino acid deficiency, had been given its name. Markovitz's husband, a mathematics professor at the university, died one year later from a heart condition that could have been brought on by the tragedy. She has remarried. But at Children's Hospital, Rosalyn Markovitz was not alone.

"Frequently, the people I meet as I go room to room just want to talk," says volunteer Alexis Vahanian. "I remember not too long ago I was in a room with a couple whose son had just been diagnosed with cancer—he was about four years old. I don't know when they were told, but I have a feeling it was that very morning. They were just talking and talking and talking. I think they were in such shock that they didn't know what else to do but talk. I just stood there and listened."

Vahanian works at Children's Hospital one day a week, spreading the word about the availability of the patient representative to newly admitted families. She distributes brochures and encourages reticent parents to voice their complaints. With the competition for the health-care dollar at an all-time high, Children's Hospital is ready and willing to extend itself by appointing people to represent the customer in order to assure customer satisfaction. Though Vahanian is not being paid, Joan Shames, under whom she works, has been employed as patient representative for more than five years.

We step off of the elevator on 10, the infant floor. Having first visited the Admissions Office, Vahanian has compiled a list of patients admitted since her rounding last week. She consults the list, then walks quickly down the hall. "A lot of these mothers seem to be so lonely up here and isolated. I think it's because they can't send the child off to the playroom, and they're sort of stuck in the room all day with the baby, where they can't associate with the other parents."

Often, conversations with parents are brief and to the point. In the first room we visit, a six-month-old baby is screaming and squirming on the father's lap. Vahanian introduces herself, quickly explains the role of the patient representative—to act as a patient advocate—and hands him a brochure. "I don't have any problems," the father says, lifting his child into the air and smiling. "You hear her? Last month, she couldn't scream at all."

Down the hall, a mother tells us, "My baby wasn't doing so well. There was something bothering her, and I couldn't pinpoint it. The doctors weren't listening to me. I kept calling the people at the clinic [the Walk-In Clinic is adjacent to the Emergency Room], and I explained everything over the phone to them, again and again. But they wouldn't believe me until I brought her in. When they realized that I was telling the truth, they admitted her."

"So what was the diagnosis?"

"She has low-grade pneumonia."

"They thought you were a hysterical mother," Vahanian says.

In another room, we meet a heavyset middle-aged woman with short-cropped steel-gray hair, who says, "After twenty-five years, I'm a parent again."

"This is your baby?" Vahanian asks incredulously.

"It is now. My daughter ran off and left her with me. Haven't seen or heard from her in a month."

Later, a father says of his thirteen-year-old daughter, "A virus attacked her brain and spinal cord and caused seizures. But her body fought it off, and now we can go home, and she'll never be back here again."

"Because you are dissatisfied here? You've had problems?"

"Because," he says, "I am not about to allow her to get sick like this again. I mean it," the father insisted. "I won't have it."

We walk into another room.

"Don't worry. They're not going to poke you," the mother says to her child.

"I didn't think they would," the little girl replies. "They don't have on white jackets."

The father comes out of the bathroom, a short man with a gigantic belly and a thick black beard. Vahanian tells the father about the patient representative, Joan Shames, and how Joan will be happy to take care of them anytime they have a problem.

"She's a nice person," Vahanian informs him.

"Yeah," says the father, "but will she pay our bill?"

One floor down, we meet a little boy, Andy, a heart transplant recipient, who has returned to the hospital after six months at home. Initially, Andy was fortunate—the wait for the organ was brief, and the transplant surgery went very smoothly. But after he went home, the usual combination of immunosuppressive medications (which transplant recipients have to take regularly for the remainder of their lives) proved ineffective. With his new heart showing signs of rejection by the body into which it had been placed, Andy has been summoned for a treatment of a special high-powered antirejection drug known as OKT-3.

If the medication does its job, Andy will be able to go back home—at least for the time being. Rejection will remain an ever-looming threat. If it turns out that OKT-3 is not the answer to Andy's rejection problem, then perhaps another heart—retransplantation—will be the only remaining option. Andy's mother tells Vahanian that she is not yet considering the alternatives, "because I know, I feel it in my bones, that this OKT-3 is going to work."

Next we meet Mrs. Lumbrowsky, from Erie, Pennsylvania, who can speak firsthand about the trauma and danger of retransplantation because her son, Eric, has received two liver transplants over the past fourteen days. "I'm glad to get it all over with at the same time," Mrs. Lumbrowsky says jokingly, although her lips tremble and her eyes tear when she smiles.

Vahanian tells her about the liver support group, for parents of children with liver disease, which happens to be meeting that evening on the floor. Mrs. Lumbrowsky says she might attend.

A young mother in the room next door says she will definitely be at the liver support group's meeting, because she's lonely and doesn't know what to do with herself. Her little daughter is dying of liver disease, and they are waiting for a matching organ to become available.

"She has biliary atresia?" asks Vahanian, referring to the liver disease that most commonly affects children. Vahanian has recognized the ailment without looking at the patient's chart, and the mother raises her eyebrows, impressed. "How did you know that?"

Indeed, it is surprising to some people that this attractive, conservatively dressed suburbanite, Alexis Vahanian, would know anything about liver disease—or any complicated and potentially fatal ailment—and the agony that parents and children endure within the walls of this pediatric institution. But as you walk the corridors of Children's Hospital, you recognize immediately that suffering is not exclusive to any group.

In 1981, Alexis Vahanian's eleven-month-old son died at Children's Hospital of biliary atresia. Back then, liver transplantation was an unproven experiment and therefore not an option. Four years after her son died, Vahanian, frustrated and lonely, felt ready to return to Children's Hospital to attempt to help other parents trapped in similar circumstances. She decided to form a liver support group, and it was this same group that she was now recommending to another mother.

"Why do I do it after what I have been through? My husband asks me that all the time, because he had the opposite reaction," Alexis

Vahanian says. "He felt that he never could come back to Children's, and he never has. Not because he dislikes the hospital or was dissatisfied with the staff, it's just that he doesn't want to be reminded of what happened.

"But many people whose children have died here come back because they feel a special closeness to their child within these walls. This was the last place their child was alive, and they got a lot of support from the staff when they were in here. When you come back, it's helpful, comforting, a way of dealing with your grief."

Vahanian has also served as a member of the Children's Hospital Bereavement Committee. All the parents whose children have died in the hospital in the recent past are invited to gather at a location outside the hospital for help through the difficult grieving process.

"These are people in the first six months of bereavement, and they've got a lot of problems. They have other children at home; they've got relatives to contend with who may not understand. There are dads who have to return to work and pretend that life is back to normal. This is an opportunity to come and say, 'Hey, I'm really still devastated. I still go to the cemetery and talk to my child.' These are things that people who haven't lost a child will probably think are kind of crazy, but for us, they are real normal.

"You get up in the middle of the night and talk to your child's picture," says Alexis Vahanian. "Over the holidays, you send out Christmas cards and put a little dot on them near your signature, symbolic of your missing child." The first Thanksgiving and Christmas are particularly difficult for the grieving parent, not only because of the pervading feeling of emptiness but also because of the misdirected sensitivities of the extended family. The general reluctance to talk about the missing child "represents kind of a double hurt to the parent. Many parents decide to stay in bed all day."

Oncology social worker Betsy Sachs served as the first group leader for parents participating in Bereavement Committee meetings. "There was one evening that was chilling, when they talked about the possessions of the dead children, and how the siblings wanted those possessions, and didn't take care of them the same way as the children who died, and how hurtful that was to the parents." The siblings also have a terrible time, however. "They can't go to their mothers and fathers for help, and their friends and teachers don't understand what they're going through.

"The other thing that I remember that was particularly poignant was their discussions about seeing the tombstone for the first time, with the name etched on it, which really made everything terribly final. That child is really dead. 'This is reality, goddam it.' "

Inevitably the parents' thoughts will turn to guilt, according to pediatrician Joel Frader, associate director of the University of Pittsburgh Center for Medical Ethics. "Family members find ways to feel responsible for the illness or incident that led to the death." Parental guilt involves a sense of having failed the child even when there was no way to prevent the event leading to the child's death, as in the still mysterious SIDS (sudden infant death syndrome). Stories such as those related by Bogeman and Beckwith, physicians who write frequently about SIDS, are not uncommon. One parent fantasized to physicians at the Seattle SIDS Center, "I told everyone that I had smothered her [my daughter] sometime during the night."

Frader says that in situations where one parent has been caring for a child when an accident occurs, the absent parent harbors angry feelings toward the allegedly negligent parent. "A father told us that his desire was to put his wife's hand into the house's main electrical supply as a punishment for her 'allowing' their son to be accidentally electrocuted in the bathtub." Many months of therapy were required to help the father sort out his thoughts and understand the fruitlessness of vengeful feelings.

Alexis Vahanian says that no matter how much time passes, how well her other two children are doing, how often she walks the corridors at Children's, how many parents and families she consults with, the same question still whirls around in her head: Why? Why is she still walking around, healthy and energetic at thirty-five, when her child was denied the opportunity to experience life?

Part III

The Pediatricians' Pediatricians

Chapter 11

"YOU'RE almost seventeen, right? What brings you to see me?" asks forty-two-year-old Carlton (Carl) Gartner. His reference to age is not meant as an inference that his new patient would be more suited to treatment at an adult health-care facility than at a children's hospital, although mature teenagers might, at times, feel uncomfortable in an atmosphere shared with infants, toddlers, and preadolescents.

The boy, whose name is Jonathan and who is very tall and thin, not quite emaciated, with long blond hair, nods and inhales deeply. His Adam's apple bobs in his long neck as he leans forward and swallows, before replying in a voice almost too gravelly for his tender age.

"Every day," he says, "without fail, I get this sharp pain in my back. At least that's the way it was before, at the beginning, six or eight months ago. But now the pain is on the move, has come around to my stomach. That's about it," he says, shrugging, "except that I am also getting chest pains." He adds, motioning with his thumb to his chest, as he leans back into his chair, "It also hurts sometimes around the heart."

Jonathan is sitting across from Gartner at one corner of an old and battered desk, while his mother, whose hair is also long, but dark, is sitting at the other corner. The family lives in a small town about sixty miles east of the hospital. Children's, only one of three pediatric institutions in the state of Pennsylvania, will normally attract patients from within a radius of 150 miles.

Jonathan and his mother have been referred by a former Children's Hospital resident who had served a three-week rotation with Gartner and his associates, Basil Zitelli, Jeffrey Malatack, and Andrew Urbach (GZMU, pronounced Gizmu), known as the pediatricians' pediatricians. The term symbolizes the inevitable, impending reality of pediatric health care: the fact that in the tertiary-care hospital the medical world is becoming too complicated and demanding for the average community doctor. Bumps, bruises, warts, colds, coughs, and other easily treatable maladies will always fall under the friendly umbrella of the private pediatrician, but when the symptoms indicate the need for care or consultation from one or more subspecialists, a knowledgeable and influential "generalist" to coordinate and control the situation is a medical must.

With the combined experience of four generations, and ranging in age from seventy to twenty-seven, the pediatricians' pediatricians will not only confirm (or question) the referring pediatrician's diagnosis, but more important, they will cut through the red tape to get the necessary subspecialist (neurologist, psychologist, oncologist, endocrinologist) for consultation—on the spot. This is the key value of the pediatricians' pediatricians, the fact that their involvement provides continuity for the family facing multisystem physical and psychosocial problems. With GZMU acting as ombudsmen, fragmentation of care by subspecialists concerned only for "their" organ systems is eliminated. When diagnosis and treatment are established—or ended—patient and family (with rare exceptions) will return to their community doctor.

In 1987, the pediatricians' pediatricians were responsible for 1,550 outpatient appointments and 806 hospital admissions, with 272 separate diagnoses, including such rare disorders as Klippel-Trenaunay-Weber syndrome (an anomaly sometimes associated with localized gigantism), Wilson's disease (an accumulation of copper in the liver), diabetes insipidus (an endocrine system disorder), and purulent pericarditis (when the membranous, fluid-filled sac surrounding the heart becomes pus-filled and infected).

Gartner, Jeffrey Malatack, Andrew Urbach, and the group's newest associate, twenty-seven-year-old Rob McGregor, as well as the semiretired founder of the group, seventy-year-old Paul Gaffney, were all chief inpatient residents (an honored fourth-year residency position for superior clinicians) at Children's, whereas Basil Zitelli served as both chief inpatient and chief outpatient pediatrics resident at Johns Hopkins University in Baltimore. In high school, Gartner had considered becoming a priest in the Jesuit order, and later he had thought seriously of internal medicine, but a summer in Haiti as a junior medical student, caring for children with basic physical disorders caused most often by nutritional deficiencies, led him to pediatrics, a calling more suited to his personality and primary interests.

"The first thing is," Jonathan's mother tells Gartner, "he can't gain weight, no matter how hard he tries and how much he eats. He just keeps getting taller—he's grown nine inches over the past eighteen months—and skinnier."

"How much do you actually eat?" asks Gartner.

"It's incredible," says his mother. "He's always hungry."

"I don't eat breakfast and lunch," Jonathan adds. "But I eat about five dinners a day."

Gartner, whose thick black brush of a mustache somewhat compensates for a lack of chin, listens carefully, nodding and making periodic notes on the index card in front of him, until the mother finishes discussing her son's overzealous eating habits. "Before we go further," he says, "I want to take a few minutes to go backward. I want to start with Jonathan's health, let's arbitrarily say, at three years of age. Was he pudgy? Chronically ill? Did he have prolonged hospitalizations? Tell me everything you remember. Spare no detail."

For the next twenty minutes, Gartner sat back and listened as the mother, with Jonathan piping in from time to time, outlined her son's medical background, naming normal childhood diseases, broken bones, visits to hospital emergency rooms. Much of the information provided by the mother and son was of intellectual rather than practical interest, but Gartner knew that the most modern medical technology available at Children's or at any high-acuity pediatric center is worthless without an accurate diagnosis. History, combined with physical assessment, was the key to diagnosis, as Gartner had learned from his mentor, Paul Gaffney, who had invited him into the practice in 1977.

Gaffney, Gartner had told me, had been preceded in this role of the generalist by Edmond McCluskey, medical director of Children's Hospital in the late 1940s. Over the years, McCluskey had seen a number of complicated referral patients in his private office, more as a favor to friends and/or colleagues than as a service to the community. As medical director of Children's Hospital, McCluskey had the influence to call in whatever subspecialists were necessary at a moment's notice, but his real genius was in administration, delegating authority and selecting members of his medical staff to help create departments and programs for the future. When McCluskey was appointed dean of the University of Pittsburgh Medical School, he drafted Gaffney to continue and expand his practice.

Although Gaffney's field was hematology, McCluskey and others had recognized a brilliance in his ability to diagnose complicated problems, based primarily on an exceedingly thorough patient history combined with a meticulous physical examination. "Paul wouldn't come out of a room and tell you, 'Well, you know, last month in this journal I read about this problem . . . ,' " said Gartner.

Gaffney would come out of the room, Gartner and other colleagues remembered, and he'd be thinking. He'd sometimes wander aimlessly through the corridors of the old hospital; he'd sit down and shake his head and cluck his tongue and cogitate—and then come up with the answer, sometimes like magic. "Anytime he made a minor error, it would be because something in the physical exam or history pushed him in the wrong direction, not because of something in a book that he read—though he was very well read. Remember," said Gartner, "and this is something that everyone tends to forget, that any well-trained subspecialist can treat an illness once the diagnosis is established. The challenge is usually in determining the problem, not in determining the treatment."

Gaffney, said Gartner, was also at his best when determining when a problem did not exist. "I remember a child who was having a third biopsy on a tongue lesion." None of the specialists could explain what was causing the repeated recurrence of the lesion, "what bizarre tumor process was taking place. And so they finally asked the great Paul Gaffney to go see this child.

"Paul looked at the child, took a history, found out about his background, found out what was going on at home, the psychosocial situation, and told those specialists right off, 'The boy is doing this to himself. Quit biopsying it. Get a counselor in here to sort out the problems. This is a fictitious lesion.' Initially, they didn't believe him," said Gartner, "but they did take his advice and call in a social worker. Weeks later, it was determined that Gaffney had been right."

Gartner leans forward, his elbows concealing the index card, now filled on both sides with hastily scribbled notes. "Did you ever notice," he asks Jonathan, "that the pain is coming on when you get a drink of water while you're working?"

Jonathan had explained that he worked during the summers and weekends, helping a construction crew. After considering Gartner's question, he replies that his pain goes away at night and comes on again in the middle of the day, not necessarily when he is drinking water.

"What do you do when you get the pain?" says Gartner.

"I keep doing what I'm doing," says Jonathan, shrugging at Gartner's question, as if to say, "What else should I do?"

The mother interrupts. "To be truthful with you, doctor, he has been pushing himself with the pain. He refuses to back off." Jonathan, who seems to be growing increasingly irritated at his mother's continued interruptions, glares across the room. "That really isn't absolutely true. You're making things look worse than they are."

"I am trying to present the doctor with an accurate portrait, Jonathan." She turns back to Gartner and hands him an envelope. "Two weeks ago he had a chest X-ray, a sonogram on his kidney, and a CAT scan. These are the results."

Gartner opens the envelope and produces a sheet of paper, which he holds up in the air and begins reading in his very distinctive manner, with the paper perhaps three inches from his right eye. As a child he had strabismus (crossed eyes), and even after corrective surgery, as with many other children, he never developed stereoscopic vision. In time, he got nearsighted in one eye.

"When I went for glasses, the ophthalmologist said, 'It's kind of silly for me to put a big, thick lens on your right eye, because you only use it for reading anyway. Anytime you look at a distance, your main image comes from your left eye.' So I read close. I used to tell people in college, especially when I got my studying done early, that my special eye allowed me to read both pages of a book at the same time. For a while, they actually believed me."

Gartner hands the report back to the mother. "Reports are fine—although this shows nothing remarkable. But for me to make a fair determination, I must see all the X-rays personally and share them with people—radiologists—with experience in pediatrics. The tests were taken," he adds, "and analyzed, in an adult hospital. Jonathan may look like an adult . . ." Gartner pauses and the mother nods.

"I'll have them send everything to you," the mother says. "I'll call first thing tomorrow."

Suddenly and abruptly Gartner changes the tone and direction of the conversation, as if shifting from first to second gear, by asking the mother about problems in the family related to either Jonathan or his siblings. The mother explains that there are four daughters, two of whom are chemically dependent, one with drugs, the other an alcoholic.

Gartner nods but does not comment. He stands up and leads Jonathan and his mother into the outer office. The mother goes outside to the waiting area, while Gartner escorts Jonathan into one of the examination rooms to have his vitals recorded by the GZMU nurse, Jan Kelchner-Cheng. He then retrieves the mother from the waiting room and leads her back into the office, explaining, "We ought to have a talk now."

With the door closed and the mother situated in the same corner seat, Gartner says, as a kind of preamble, that he doesn't want her to think that he is prying, but he needs to understand the details of all aspects of Jonathan's life in order to try to unravel the mystery of the disease that may well be afflicting him.

The mother has obviously been expecting the conversation, for she launches into the discussion without hesitation. "Our lives are pretty screwed-up right now, doctor. We've had a lot of things happen to us—serious things. And Jonathan, he's what I call a 'stuffer.' Keeps everything inside."

They talk a little bit about her chemically dependent children, but she presses on to something else that is obviously bothering her. "It must have been a year and a half ago. He was helping a friend take apart a car, and the friend's mother would always be watching over them down in their garage. That was reasonable enough, but after a while Jonathan started getting these secret-admirer letters, and those letters became upsetting to me and to him as well. Jonathan is kind, however, and didn't want to say anything to his friend or even to the mother about the letters, but they just kept coming."

Jonathan's mother looks up at Gartner and shakes her head. "Don't ask me why we didn't put a stop to this when the letters continued. Or when she would call him up on the telephone or come to our house to visit, but Jonathan insisted that he wanted to handle the problem himself, in his own way. This was the mother of his good friend. He didn't want to hurt or embarrass his friend. We waited for something to happen—I mean for Jonathan to do something about the situation or for the situation to just play itself out, but last month, when she came to visit him at home again, we decided we had had enough. We went to the police, explained the situation, and insisted that the mother get psychiatric treatment over this fixation.

"At the same time all of this was happening," the mother continues, "Jonathan's long-time girlfriend met another guy, a weight-lifter. All the while, Jonathan was growing sicker, and he was losing muscle mass and getting skinnier. The weightlifter probably just started to look a little better. She broke up with Jonathan three weeks ago." The mother pauses and looks across the desk at Gartner. "Jonathan really loved that girl. All the money he ever made on his part-time jobs he spent on her." The mother smiles sadly. "I guess that's about it."

"Do you think he's into drugs or alcohol at all?" Gartner asks.

"I don't think so," says the mother. "He's seen what his sisters have had happen to them. Their lives are terrible, to put it mildly."

"And how do you and your husband get along?"

The mother catches her breath—in fact, she almost chokes—but she answers with a sad smile. "We get along okay these days, but we've had plenty of problems through our lives, as you can imagine."

"Did Jonathan's pain intensify as his problems with his girlfriend—or with the friend's mother—increased?"

"Jonathan has been especially depressed," said the mother, "that doctors have been unable to diagnose his problem. He can't understand it. I mean, you people are supposed to know. . . ."

"We're supposed to know a lot of things that we actually do not know," says Gartner. "Doctors, after all, are only human—most of us, anyway," he adds as kind of a joke to himself.

"Jonathan gets in his car and drives around every night. He varies from deep, glum moods to out-and-out anger. His grades have gone down. He used to be a top student; now he's failing English. He used to have a photographic memory; now he can't remember very many things at all. He does go to school regularly, however. He doesn't like to miss."

Once again, Gartner thanks the mother, escorts her into the waiting area, and heads to the examination room to see Jonathan. On his way, he is stopped in the corridor by one of his partners, Jeffrey Malatack, who wants to talk about an interesting patient—a little boy from Guatemala—with extra digits on his hands and feet. The foster mother, who lives sixty miles from Pittsburgh, had asked Malatack to conduct a thorough physical examination on the child, who has arrived in this country within the past month.

Malatack explains that he originally met this woman at Continuity Clinic—essentially a free clinic at Children's in which pediatric residents treat and follow patients who do not have their own community pediatrician. Each GZMU partner will help "precept" residents serving at this clinic once each week. "She's over fifty years old, has already raised two adopted families, the first as a relatively young woman. That family is grown. Now she's started over again with young kids, primarily with serious medical problems. When I met her, she had just become a foster parent to a Central American baby, half Indian, half black, born in a barroom, probably with fetal alcohol syndrome. I told her," said Malatack, "if she could do this for needy children, then I could be her doctor for free." In addition to the extra fingers and toes, there's something else, Malatack tells Gartner. "See if a syndrome hits you," Malatack says.

Gartner follows Malatack into the examination room. The boy is dark and exotic-looking with long black hair, big knobby knees, short arms. Gartner wonders aloud to Malatack about dwarfism.

"He looks very small, but he will be five in December," the mother, heavyset, smiling, and gray-haired, says. She adds, "I can't say the Spanish word for hurt, but don't be afraid of hurting him. If you're too rough, he knows the word, 'Ow!' "

Concentrating, Gartner listens to the heart through the stethoscope for a very long time. "Obvious heart disease," he says softly.

Malatack nods, as Gartner gingerly examines the digits on the child's hands and feet, which are broad and flat, with hypoplastic (undeveloped) nails. Looking up at Malatack, he comments: "Possible Rubenstein-Taybi?"

"Let's go see," Malatack says. "I'll be back," he tells the mother as they exit the room.

Malatack heaves a thick reference book, entitled *Recognizable Patterns of Human Malformation*, out of his bookcase, dumps it on his desk, and begins flipping through pages, as Gartner peers over his shoulder. In my month with GZMU and nearly two years at One Children's Place, I was always surprised—and pleased—to see doctors consult the literature for basic information and verification.

"He has fingers that look like that," says Gartner, pointing down at an enlarged photograph of a child with Rubenstein-Taybi, "but it's not exactly the same."

"He's really something," says Malatack, shaking his head. "We should bring in [pediatric cardiologist] Jay Fricker, as well as [geneticist] Mark Steele. See what they can tell us."

Gartner agrees, and after a few minutes of additional discussion, tells Malatack to keep him informed. He retraces his steps down the hall toward the examination room where Jonathan has been waiting. As we walk, Gartner says of his own patient, "This is very serious. I don't take this lightly at all. Whenever you have a chronic pain of that magnitude, you have some major physical problem or some serious emotional dysfunction. Either way, it must be confronted—and quickly."

As the examination begins, Jonathan, who has stripped down to his underwear, says, "Please don't touch my feet. I'm very ticklish." You can see that he is attempting to hold back his laughter. Even the thought of Gartner touching his feet makes him want to giggle.

"Do you smoke?" asks Gartner, as the examination begins.

"Yes."

"I know this is a sore subject, but do you use drugs or alcohol?"

"Not anymore," Jonathan answers. "I did when I was twelve or thirteen." He adds, "That's probably why I smoke so much—maybe one and a half packs a day. It helps me out. Gives me something to do. Takes the tension away from not using, when my friends are doing the drugs and I'm around them."

Just as he did with Jonathan's mother, Gartner nods somewhat impassively. He does not want to lead Jonathan to believe that he is passing judgment on him one way or the other. "Do you have a girlfriend?" he asks.

"She's dead," says Jonathan.

"You mean you broke up?"

"Yes. That's what I mean."

"Pretty rough time for you, I imagine?" says Gartner.

"For a little while, but now it's okay."

There is a long silence now and Gartner proceeds with the examination. He is especially careful, warning Jonathan in advance, when touching the boy's feet. Gartner needs to touch the feet only to hold the leg steady in order to test reflexes, but Jonathan jumps and yelps at least a half dozen times before the maneuver can be completed. "This drives me crazy," shrieks Jonathan. For a moment in that room, he is no longer a young man with serious adult problems to cope with. He squirms and laughs like a ten-year-old, wriggling, wrestling, and having fun.

Reality returns almost immediately when Gartner completes the examination, looks up at Jonathan, and says, "I'll tell you the truth. This is going to be a tough one to figure out."

Back in his office with Jonathan and his mother, he tells them that before they do anything else, he wants to look at all the X-rays and the results of all the other tests that have been done. "There's a condition that has a real funny name, and that's 'beer drinker's kidney' (urethrapelvic junction obstruction). Every time you drink a lot of liquid, you get a lot of pain. This could be it, but I'm not sure."

He looks at the mother. "His exam is normal. He's not wasted or emaciated or anything like that; he's just a normal growing adolescent boy whose weight is not keeping up with his height. After I examine the tests and X-rays, I'll contact you. Maybe we can figure out a way of getting him into our Emergency Room in order to X-ray him at the point when his pain is actually occurring."

Gartner returns to his office after Jonathan and his mother have departed and sinks back into an old swivel chair behind his desk. "He's got abdominal pain, which is a common symptom in children, but it's an atypical abdominal pain. Usually the child is a little younger, nine to twelve, and it is associated with pallor, although not fatigue or weight loss. And the pain is central in the abdomen. His pain, conversely, is distinctly flank. Even Appley, the great British pediatrician, says in his book on recurrent abdominal pain in children, 'Be leery of pain which is at an unusual location outside the central abdomen.'

"To top it off," says Gartner, "this kid's got a horrible home situation; he's got drug addiction and a stressed family and a breakup with his girlfriend, so it may be that this pain is just his coping pain. Instead of having a headache, he has pain in his chest or flank—or wherever. This is a situation where I'm going to have to see him a couple of times; talk with him some more. Examine him, watch his weight gain, weight loss. I'm not sure I'm going to put him through any other tests right now—unless the pain becomes more severe or changes in location."

At this moment, Malatack appears in the doorway to announce the Guatemalan boy's diagnosis, which he had eventually determined and then confirmed with Fricker and Steele. "It's Ellis-van Creveld syndrome," a congenital syndrome typified among other symptoms by extra fingers and toes, and congenital heart defects, which was the aspect most worrisome to Malatack. "He has holes in the two upper chambers of his heart, which are easily fixable, if it isn't too late." By "too late" Malatack means that the defects might now be or will soon become irreparable, thus leading to the child's early death.

"It's such a shame," says Malatack, who has been described by his partner Andrew Urbach as "the civil libertarian of the group, externally more volatile than the rest of us," the person most apt to take up the cause of the underdog. Malatack, in his late thirties, is married with five children. He grew up in a coal-mining town in eastern Pennsylvania, where, although his parents are no longer living, he periodically returns to catch up with his past.

"This kid would not need to be here at all if he had had the proper medical treatment in the first place in his own country," Malatack says. "But now even his teeth are rotting." He shakes his head and kicks at an imaginary speck on the carpet. "Sometimes the whole damn health-care system makes you sick," he says. "Here we are in Pittsburgh, with the largest pediatric liver transplant program in the world, spending upwards of $200,000 per procedure— a hundred times every year—when we are confronted by this lack of basic medical care in most of the rest of the world. I'm telling you, something has to be done about this. These situations can't go on as they are now. It just doesn't make sense; it simply doesn't seem right."

Chapter 12

PEDIATRIC resident Laurie Penix, currently serving a three-to-four-week rotation with GZMU, is shaking her head and tssking away as she examines an X-ray on the backlighted screen, "which," she says, "shows a four-month-old named Aaron wth a liver mass [tumor]." Continuing to mumble about the inequities of life, Penix, who has conducted a thorough physical examination of the child, now summons Gartner. He has already viewed the X-ray, which was sent in advance by the referring pediatrician. Together, carrying the X-ray with them, they enter the examination room to meet and talk with the family.

In response to Gartner's first question about whether she has noticed anything different about her child, the mother replies, "The last couple of days it seemed like he wasn't really drinking a full bottle. He was eating the same amount, but just in more numerous increments."

Gartner pauses and peers at the mother. He speaks softly but directly. "We don't know exactly what is going on, but this will be a difficult day for you. I know that for certain."

Immediately, the mother starts to cry.

"I know you're worried," says Gartner, "but we aren't going to hide anything from you. You should know how it is."

The father is standing in the background with his arms folded, his face a stiff and unresponsive mask. A sister of the mother's who is a nurse, on hand for technical guidance and moral support, is sitting side by side with the mother, holding her hand. Gartner repeats his initial statement two or three times. "This is going to be a very difficult day, but I want to assure you that you'll be the first to know whatever we find out. Nothing will be kept from you, that's a promise."

Meanwhile, Gartner has been slowly familiarizing and ingratiating himself with little Aaron. "You're a smily guy," he says. At first he pulls the child's diaper back for a better view of the abdominal area but then has second thoughts about that particular tactic. "Let's protect ourselves from sneak attack," he jokes. Everybody laughs. As he presses lightly on each part of the abdominal area, he continues a running commentary, which seems to have a calming effect on both family and child. Finally, he looks up at Penix: "Left upper abdomen seems empty. There's definitely a mass on the other side."

Now Gartner turns on the X-ray screen and inserts the film so that he can explain the problem and field any questions. On the glass, they see the outline of the kidney and the liver, a clear delineation of both organs, but on top of the liver, a big black threatening mass. "You can see the liver," he says, pointing, "and then those black cysts. Those are the worrisome things—those cysts." The parents soon turn away from the screen and stare at the child; the sister nods in Gartner's direction, although she too seems somewhat dazed.

Gartner says, "What's the worst thing you can worry about? A cancerous liver tumor, that's the worst thing. The best treatment is total removal. At this point, I would just say to you to keep an open mind. We have to conduct a number of tests before coming to any conclusions. We'll do a CT [computerized tomography] scan today"—Gartner looks over to Penix—"and a biopsy [excision of a small piece of the tumor, for microscopic examination] tomorrow.

"If the tumor happens to be benign," he says, "we will present the baby to the Tumor Board." This is a group of radiologists, surgeons, and oncologists, Gartner later explained, on top of national trends in cancer treatment, who meet weekly to discuss and examine the best possible therapy for each patient. As a matter of practice, GZMU will consult the board as often as possible. "They may decide to recommend that the tumor be taken out, even though it isn't cancerous. But first things first—and that's the next test."

He then provides directions to the Admissions Office. "They're already waiting. They'll take care of you when you get there."

As Gartner smiles and begins to walk out of the room, the sister leans over to the mother and whispers, "He looks like Dad."

The same day that little Aaron was examined in the GZMU offices, Penix and Gartner also met Melissa for the first time, an eight-year-old girl who, upon experiencing repeated back pain and increasing leg stiffness, had been taken by her parents to a chiropractor. Soon after—two weeks ago—she suddenly lost her ability to walk.

"This case is perplexing," Gartner tells one of his partners, Andrew Urbach, who is also seeing patients that afternoon. "She giggles; she's happy, even though she hasn't been able to move her legs. But she's real inconsistent. Sometimes she feels me [stimulate her skin], sometimes she doesn't. Sometimes she has pain. Sometimes she has reflexes. Sometimes the reflexes are on the left, and sometimes they're on the right. The only way you can make her respond predictably is when you sneak up on her and prick her with a pin. But she's awful young," says Gartner, "awful young for 'conversion.' "

Gartner is referring to a "conversion reaction," a common problem in pediatrics, defined by *Taber's Cyclopedic Medical Dictionary* as "a type of hysterical neurosis in which there is loss or alteration in physical functioning suggesting a physical disorder, but instead representing the expression of a psychological conflict or need. The disturbance is not under a voluntary control."

Urbach and Gartner momentarily discuss the need to be especially thorough in this situation because of the legal and moral ramifications of making a mistake. Assuming that a serious and significant physical problem is "in the mind" and discovering later that the problem did indeed exist could be personally and professionally devastating.

"But she's too darn young," repeats Gartner. "She's only eight, which means that we have no choice but to conduct the most thorough of physical examinations. In fact, my fear is that it may well be a spinal cord lesion. If this is true, and we don't follow up on the possibility, in another couple of weeks there's no question that she will never walk again."

"I wonder," said Urbach, "if the chiropractor traumatized her in some way."

Gartner shrugs. "She did walk into his office, but she couldn't walk out."

"What puzzles me," says Penix, who has been listening intently to the conversation, "is why the parents waited for two weeks to do something for a child who suddenly couldn't walk. I'm certain that their actions were not malicious, but it just boggles my mind how thoughtless people can sometimes be."

Gartner decides to ask a neurologist to conduct an immediate emergency examination—a natural next step. Within an hour, a neurologist has examined Melissa, who tells Gartner he also suspects the likelihood of a spinal cord lesion, and Melissa is sent to the nearby Nuclear Magnetic Resonance (NMR) Center for confirmation of diagnosis.

During an evaluation of a respiratory infection, five-year-old Joseph Jacobs received a chest X-ray at his local hospital, which revealed the existence of a tumor. Jeffrey Malatack suspects it to be a neuroblastoma, a dangerous type of malignancy chiefly occurring in infants and children in the chest and abdominal areas. Malatack says that the hospital in which Jacobs was initially examined took a larger X-ray than normal, especially in the abdominal area, because of inexperience in the process of X-raying children. "They inadvertently got a shot of the belly, at which point they accidentally discovered the tumor." The discovery, from Malatack's point of view, was a mixed blessing.

"Sometimes, we suspect, tumors like this in young children resolve themselves by maturation, and we don't even catch them. But now because we know it exists, we will have to put this family through a whole lot of trouble, when it might have gone away all by itself." In response to the idea of extending all X-rays into the abdominal areas, he explained that it would be inadvisable to expose children to low-level radiation even on the chance of finding a tumor, because it's a million-to-one chance and the tumor will very often self-destruct anyway.

Bertram R. Girdany, director of the Hillman Center for Children's Radiology, explained that pediatric radiologists are equipped with special equipment, such as filters, screens, and faster film, to minimize the possibility of overexposure to diagnostic radiation. There are also "gentle restraints" for children undergoing X-ray to keep them immobilized. "One of the surprising things is that children usually fall asleep once they are secure. Children want security; they don't want to flop all over the place."

Girdany says that many parents do not understand that interpreting X-ray films of children requires specialized knowledge. "The old cliché, which I hate to use, that children are not small adults, still applies. Children have their own diseases; children are growing. Their bones are often irregular," unlike regular adult formations. "They have different acute illnesses. They have different kinds of tumors. They have different manifestations of allergies and a whole series of illnesses that are peculiar to them.

"Over the past few years," says Girdany, "there have been a whole mess of imaging techniques introduced into radiology, beginning with CT," which involves heavier doses of radiation but at the same time permits a wide cross section of views of the human body. "In a standard X-ray picture, we can see basically four densities: the densities of air, of fat, of most soft tissues (including blood), and of bone. Or we can use a contrast material like barium—so that gives us five densities. By using CT, the radiologist can examine an area in a thousand different dimensions. The newest imaging technique, nuclear magnetic resonance, provides even more depth, says Girdany, who prefers ultrasound whenever possible, because it is the safest of all available diagnostic avenues. It does not use radiation. It uses sonar, which, he admits, has one drawback: "It cannot be used effectively in the GI tract or in the lungs"—anywhere with air. "The rays seem to bounce off; you get a very bright image but no detail."

Unfortunately, the importance of providing children with special attention will not register on some of the residents who pass through the Radiology Department from local hospitals in a three-month rotation in general diagnostic radiology. Pediatric radiology requires one to two years of specialized training, according to Girdany, one of the first pediatric radiologists in the world. (Today, there are about a thousand members of the Society of Pediatric Radiology, of which Girdany was a charter member.)

Sitting side by side with Girdany, Malatack examines newly developed X-rays of the Jacobs child. "Looks as if he has a calcified mass—a suprarenal—which is separate from the kidney."

Girdany agrees but is disturbed. "We didn't use contrast," he says, meaning that in order to see certain structures more clearly, an illuminating material is often filtered through the veins of the patient before the X-ray. He summons the resident who supervised the procedure.

"Why didn't you use contrast?"

"Well, we couldn't get the IV in. I tried, and then someone else tried, and then someone else tried after that. No one could get the IV in."

"You should have called the house doctor," Malatack says, referring to the third-year resident on call in the hospital. "That's the easiest thing to do."

"We've got plenty of people who can put in an IV," says Girdany, obviously quite unhappy with and perhaps a little embarrassed by his resident. "This is a children's hospital, for God's sake."

Although Malatack can have the X-ray repeated with contrast, he decides to turn the patient over to the Department of Surgery and let the surgeons decide what to do. He suspects that they will want to operate immediately, because judging from what he can see on the film, there is no time to waste.

As Malatack heads back to 7 North, he passes the Department of Cardiology, glancing down the corridor toward the laboratory where the Guatemalan boy for whom he has shown such concern will soon be undergoing a cardiac catherization, a precision procedure in which a tiny plastic tube is passed into the heart through a blood vessel. Samples of blood are withdrawn for testing, while blood pressure and cardiac output are measured. Soon he will know the full extent of this little boy's problem.

Back on 7 North, at the nurses' station, Malatack is approached by a resident who explains the difficulty she experienced in performing a successful spinal tap on a patient of Malatack's. Timmy, admitted late last night, is a young boy from Johnstown, Pennsylvania, with an immune system dysfunction who presented with a fever and seizures, causing Malatack to worry that the child was suffering from spinal meningitis. "We tried six times to tap his spine," said the resident, "but we just couldn't do it."

A spinal or "lumbar" puncture (tap) is routinely performed to obtain specimens of cerebrospinal fluid (CSF), which circulates between the lower back and the brain. To retrieve the fluid and examine it for possible infection, doctors insert a long needle into the spinal canal. It's a tricky procedure because the fluid is contained in the middle layer of a three-layer lining that surrounds the spinal cord within the spinal column, but it is usually mastered during the first year of residence.

Malatack says to the resident, "When you have trouble tapping the spine, the best thing to do is to sit the patient up."

"We did sit him up a couple of times. We just couldn't seem to get it together and do it. We even called in night float," says the resident, referring to the third-year resident who serves as house doctor from 11 P.M. to 11 A.M. This month, that person is Molly O'Gorman. In fact, at this point O'Gorman appears, about to go home. In wrinkled scrubs and a Levi jacket, she says she's been up all night and she's also stiff and sore, because before coming to work, she did a twelve-mile run in preparation for an upcoming ten-kilometer race.

"I'm sorry about last night," she says, referring to the failed spinal tap. We tried and tried." Malatack nods but does not comment. "You know I'm good," she says. "It just didn't work out last night."

In the Procedures Room opposite the nurses' station on 7 North, Timmy's spine is being tapped at that moment by a newly arrived resident who was lucky enough to have gotten a full night's sleep.

Timmy's father and mother are standing at the door to Timmy's room, waiting for their son to return and also waiting for Malatack in order to talk with him. Their bodies are so stiff with fear and worry that they look like mannequins displayed in the doorway. The father stutters before he speaks; it requires four tries just to get his sentence started. "Do they have medicine to get it out of his spine if it's spinal meningitis?"

Malatack assures him that there is medication that can deal with the problem, although with Timmy's immunosuppressed state, "you try not to give them any medication that could cause complications." Malatack wants to avoid a conversation about hypotheticals, which could alarm the parents unnecessarily. He turns away abruptly, perhaps somewhat rudely, and walks out the door and down the hall to watch the final moments of the spinal tap as it is taking place. "I'll be back," he mumbles.

The resident has been successful by the time we arrive. Already the spinal fluid, the color of pink grapefruit juice, is dripping out of a puncture hole in the spine. There is about an eighth-inch sample in six separate test tubes. Meanwhile, Timmy is fighting; it's quite painful, and he is squirming on the table, screaming and crying.

With the procedure completed, we start to leave the room, but the nurse—a very young nurse—who has been helping the resident says in a very high, soft voice as she picks Timmy up, "How long is he going to make it?"

"You mean survive?" says Malatack.

"His mom and dad said yesterday they didn't think he'd make it much longer," the nurse says.

"Oh, we're going to get him better," says Malatack. "We're going to get him better. There's no doubt about that."

Later, I ask Malatack if such situations are common—nurses asking about the possible fate of their patients.

"I don't think it happens that often. Nurses usually keep their own counsel and seek information and support within their own group. She was a little bold to even say it, I thought, in all honesty, but I understood that she was trying to diffuse her own anxiety over the whole thing by talking to me about it. I have no problem with that—in fact, I think it's healthy."

Joe Jacobs' tumor was surgically removed that evening. The following morning we met with a technician in the Pathology Department to examine cells from a bone marrow sample, taken by Malatack during surgery and displayed on three separate slides, for evidence of cell immaturity—a frequent indication of neuroblastoma or malignancy. Under the microscope each cell is represented by a tiny dot. Most of them are pink but a few are purple, indicating the nucleus of a cell cluster. Malatack says they are searching for a special telltale cluster or formation of cells, a kind of "monotonous" pattern, as distinguished from the rest of the cells, and after peering silently into the microscope for a number of minutes, concentrating on each cluster of dots, which, to the naked eye, resemble fragments of a classic aboriginal sand painting, he shakes his head, sighs, and tells the pathologist who has been examining the cells with him, "I don't like those cells; I don't like those cells at all."

The pathologist nods but is unwilling to commit herself. "It's not so bad," she says. She informs Malatack that there are three slides, which will require about twenty minutes each to examine, and she will contact him the moment there is a definite determination.

Malatack walks out of the room. Then, as if a second thought has just occurred to him, he stops, turns, and pokes his head back in through the door. "Don't find anything. Please don't find anything, if you can help it."

Two hours later, the pathologist paged Malatack—Joseph Jacobs was fine.

The parents of Carl Gartner's patient, Baby Aaron, were also treated with similar good fortune the following afternoon. "After biopsy, the lesion turned out to be a benign hamartoma, which is not a tumor," said Gartner, "just a proliferation of normal tissue in the liver. It was subsequently removed surgically, and the baby's doing fine. Aaron should have a very positive long-term outlook."

Eight-year-old Melissa, the little girl who suddenly could not walk, was also extraordinarily lucky. "The results of the NMR indicated a bone tumor impinging on her spinal cord, which we thought for sure was malignant," says Gartner. "But it wasn't!

"The cyst was surgically removed. Within twenty-four hours after surgery, she was moving her toes. By the time she went home four days later, she was able to lift her knees up off the bed. I saw her this Monday, which is about two weeks post-op; she walked into the office. To go from paraplegia to walking in that short period of time is absolutely miraculous. I can't remember anybody with paraplegia, for as long as she had it, who got better as fast as she did. It's really remarkable."

Carl Gartner never saw Jonathan again after that initial interview, but he did remain in contact with the mother, who reported over the following months a gradual reduction of her son's symptoms. "Sometimes you just need moral support," says Gartner. "Sometimes a doctor can assure you that, despite how you feel about yourself or the way your life is going at any given moment, you are actually going to be all right."

Chapter 13

PROMPTLY at 8:45 A.M., Andy Urbach, Jeff Malatack, and Basil Zitelli cram into Carl Gartner's tiny office for the regular Monday morning sign-in meeting. Each weekend, on a rotating basis, one of the pediatricians' pediatricians—Zitelli on this particular weekend—assumes active responsibility for the practice, taking emergency telephone calls from patients at home and/or from nurses and doctors in the hospital, and "rounding" personally, both Saturday and Sunday, on each GZMU patient in the hospital. Missing is Rob MacGregor, who is on vacation for the next few weeks, and Paul Gaffney, who although a frequent visitor and regular consultant, no longer participates actively in the practice. Zitelli is perspiring as he begins the discussion.

"It was that bad on the weekend?" Gartner asks, handing Zitelli a tissue.

"No, it was relatively quiet. Twenty-two patients, whereas last weekend there were thirty-seven. But I played racketball this morning. Just finished a few minutes ago." Zitelli, perhaps five feet, two inches in his stocking feet, is wearing a lab coat and old-fashioned wing-tip shoes, from which he wipes the dust, after dabbing his face with Gartner's tissue.

Reading from a set of index cards, Zitelli begins by talking about an Amish boy. "Came in because of a cough," says Zitelli. "No evidence of what parents suspected: pneumonia. He'll go home today."

Zitelli's next patient is an eleven-and-a-half-month-old failure-to-thrive boy, who, according to Zitelli, lives in a "chaotic, horrendous social situation. The child has been eating like a horse since getting here. He suffers from no growth—probably because he gets no food. He's going to be in for a while," says Zitelli, shaking his head in disgust, "until we can sort out the social situation."

"The mother wants to take him home?" asks Gartner.

Zitelli nods. "But I won't let him leave the hospital."

"Are you ready for a battle?"

"Whatever it takes," says Zitelli. "I feel that we have to do something in this situation, before it's too late."

Zitelli continues with the next patient. The child was admitted Friday night with a history of fever and infection. He had gone to Kennywood (a local amusement park), where he repeatedly refused to walk. The father, a nurse, noted that his knees and ankles were hot. He took the child to the Children's Hospital Emergency Room. He was admitted, and liberal doses of Tylenol were prescribed. "The following day he was afebrile [without fever], and was able to bear weight. By Sunday he was perfectly asymptomatic, normal gait. Virus came on fast, unlike rheumatic fever." He shrugs. "Tough night for the parents."

Now Zitelli is discussing a child admitted with pertussis (whooping cough), and whether parents and siblings should also be treated because of the infectious nature of the disease. Urbach consults a reference book, reads aloud the recommendations; they decide that the entire family should be medicated as a safety precaution, a task performed later that day.

Urbach is especially soft-spoken. In fact, you have to listen consciously—kind of cock an ear in his direction—in order to hear every word he says. He is also the most casual of the group; his shoes this morning are Indian mocs. Most pediatricians found their way into this branch of medicine sometime during their medical education because they came to realize that they liked or even loved children, while enjoying the company of other pediatricians, but Urbach was one step ahead. "I can remember in ninth or tenth grade, my family visited a physician friend in the Midwest, a radiologist, and she took me to the hospital to spend the day with her. She arranged for me to see surgery, and then she said, 'What do you want to do?' I said I'd like to work in a pediatrician's office for an afternoon. I did, and I found it fascinating."

"Guess who is coming back in today," Zitelli announces. "His family ran out of money, so we are forced to re-admit him to our RCU [Respiratory Care Unit]."

Zitelli is referring to a child, John, who had cerebral palsy at birth with substantial brain injury and little residual brain function, who for a long while had required twenty-four-hour ventilator support (artificial breathing). Some months ago, John had returned to the hospital with a severe case of pneumonia, at which time GZMU was able not only to treat and subsequently cure the pneumonia but also to improve the child's condition so that he would be free of ventilator dependency—a great achievement for the doctors but a financial disaster for the foster mother (custody of the child had been relinquished by the biological mother at birth).

Malatack explained the irony of the situation: A program exists in Pennsylvania and in some other states for the home care (round-the-clock nursing, in this child's case) of technologically dependent children. (The fund represents an annual taxpayer drain of many hundreds of thousands of dollars, but it is an efficient investment, because the state would otherwise be obligated to pay two or three times as much for the exact same treatment in the hospital.) Although John was free of his ventilator, in no way was he cured; he still required full-time nursing care at home. ("His best and most normal function is that he smiles," Malatack says.) But since he was not attached to a ventilator, his mother could no longer tap into the fund for technologically dependent children, and this was why Basil Zitelli had been forced to return John to the Respiratory Care Unit at Children's.

Not that the state government would actually abandon John—or any helpless child for that matter—but an esoteric and convoluted tangle of red tape and bureaucratic protocol first had to be deciphered and then subsequently untangled in order to find a program to fit John's special circumstances. "It's possible," said Malatack, "that we could file an exception waiver," meaning that although John no longer technically requires a ventilator, he is just as dependent as those who do need ventilator support.

Malatack pointed out that John's presence in the hospital would be an inducement for the state to agree to a waiver because of the expense of hospital care compared with home care. "It's a strange game we sometimes play here, doctor against government," he said, "although in this circumstance, the odds are in the patient's favor."

Zitelli nods, but he is angry, unable to drop the subject and move on to the next patient. "The government is willing to pay $1,000 a day for a patient in our Respiratory Care Unit but not $100 a day for nursing care at home. It's crazy," he says. "It just, just . . ." He sighs, shakes his head, lowers his voice, and looks at his partners. "Well, you know. You've all been through it before, but it pisses me off every time I think about it."

There is a long silence in the room, as Urbach, Malatack, and Gartner, each of whom has experienced similar roadblocks, silently sympathize.

"This home ventilator program," says Malatack, "for all the virtues of it, has made it easy for us not to make the hard decisions that we sometimes should be forced to make. With the funds available, it is often easier for the physician to send the child home and the family to accept the child, no matter what the limitations, than to sit down and decide that saving the child's life might be a futile pursuit and shouldn't be done. Before this home ventilator care program, we were faced with hard decisions."

"I do the same thing that everyone else does," Urbach admits. "I send them home, because I don't want to make such a difficult decision."

"I still think the best answer is a continuing dialogue with the parents," says Zitelli.

"That doesn't always work," says Urbach. "I can't tell you how often I've tried it. So often the family won't listen, and if you push too hard, there's a danger that they will think you are trying to kill their child."

"If we would cut out those people who really shouldn't have it," says Malatack, referring to the children reduced to a completely vegetative state, "we would save fifty percent of the money that is allocated for home ventilator care. This means the right people— the children who can achieve a certain measure of life quality— would end up with the ventilator."

Soon after the meeting is adjourned, Basil Zitelli is paged to the Emergency Room. An hour before, he had received a call from a community pediatrician, Dr. Reynolds, about an infant who has been experiencing fits of irritability since birth. He had promised Reynolds that he would see the child as soon as he and the parents arrived. An intern introduces himself to Zitelli in the ER, explaining that he has already conducted a preliminary examination.

Although most attending physicians in the hospital are compensated on a relatively equal basis for teaching, no group in the hospital takes more seriously or assumes more regular responsibility for the education of residents than GZMU. Many pediatricians attending in the hospital must agree to supervise residents on a floor or in a ward for one month each year, but in evidence of their commitment to teaching, the pediatricians' pediatricians voluntarily serve two months each in rotation. If their dedication to teaching is commendable, many colleagues question its wisdom—at least in relation to promotion within the professorial hierarchy of the university and its related benefits of salary, recognition, and security.

Most people outside the medical world do not fully understand that each doctor employed by a university medical center—whether specialist or generalist—must simultaneously serve two masters, the university's requirement for research and the patients' need for clinical care. The University of Pittsburgh evaluates and promotes its faculty according to their scientific recognition and achievement, measured both by the papers published in prestigious journals and by the research money generated from scientific foundations and from the National Institutes of Health for current and future projects.

As an example of the importance of research in the minds of the leaders of the academic community, Thomas K. Oliver, currently the vice president of the American Board of Pediatrics, cited a list of ten priorities recently set forth by Harvard University as to what medical schools should be doing. "The first was research—advancing knowledge," said Oliver. "The tenth—and last—was educating medical students." This is especially disappointing, said Oliver, since "a number of different institutions and investigators can do research but only one particular institution—medical schools—can teach medical students."

Oliver, who was chief of Pediatric Services at Children's Hospital until his resignation, early in 1987, was succeeded in 1989 by pediatric endocrinologist Mark Sperling, originally of Melbourne, Australia, and subsequently, of the Children's Hospital Medical Center of Cincinnati. Sperling is the person responsible for the day-to-day operations of the medical staff, the selection and supervision of interns and residents, the planning of their training program, the recruitment of new faculty, and the generation of research projects and funding for both the university and the hospital. The chief of Pediatric Services at Children's also serves as the chairman of the Department of Pediatrics of the University of Pittsburgh School of Medicine, which means that he or she must walk the line between the hospital, which has a strong and enduring commitment to the community, and the university, which, as an academic institution, emphasizes scientific rather than clinical interests. Between the time Oliver resigned and Sperling came on board, GZMU coordinated most pediatric intern and resident training activities.

Now, in the ER, the intern who had interviewed the parents reiterated to Zitelli that this child, Reynolds' patient, had experienced lifelong (he is thirty-two weeks old) fits of irritability and flailing of arms and legs, occurring almost always after feeding. The parents had tried various formulas over the months for the baby, but now the fits have increased anyway. The baby, born by C-section, is also constipated. He had been treated for jaundice shortly after birth and was released from the hospital after a month. The intern tells Zitelli that he sent for the medical records but has not yet received them.

Zitelli listens carefully, then becomes a polite but relentless interrogator.

"Is the child at all consolable?" asks Zitelli.

"Yes, by holding and rocking him, you can usually calm him down, but according to his parents, not always."

"Anything that can be predicted to bring these fits on?"

"Feeding, after about two ounces," the intern replies.

"Is there anything that will make it go away?" asks Zitelli.

"When he stops eating."

"What are you thinking about?" asks Zitelli, meaning in relation to diagnosis and treatment. "What should be done next?"

"Perhaps investigate possible trauma, the history of constipation."

"What do the stools look like?" asks Zitelli.

"Dark green."

"Consistency?" asks Zitelli.

"Fairly hard."

Zitelli talks about intestinal obstruction and lectures briefly about some of the possible ramifications if such an obstruction exists. The questioning then continues. Zitelli brings up Sandifer's syndrome, which causes children to writhe and contort uncontrollably, looking as if they had some neurologic dysfunction.

"What else?" Zitelli says to the intern. "What about epilepsy?"

"It's possible. Could it be something brought on by exertion?" says the intern.

"No, a child that young doesn't exert himself enough for that." There's a long silence, during which the intern begins to look uncomfortable.

"What about growth?" asks Zitelli after a while.

The intern perks up. "That may be important."

They discuss the child's dimensions and size and decide that she's a little smaller than she ought to be.

"Her eye is remarkable," the intern then says. "She has this uncoordinated gaze, and two scratches above the forehead, which she got during one of her recent seizures."

"The pain must be pretty severe if it's caused her to scratch herself," says Zitelli. "Well, how do you think we ought to proceed? Put your nickel down. Tell me what we should do next."

The intern stares at Zitelli impassively, searching his mind for an answer. "I guess we should go into the examining room and introduce you to the parents and the child."

In the room, the mother begins a long discourse on all the different formulas they've tried in order to change or alter this pattern of irritability.

"Describe an episode," says Zitelli.

The father says, "She'll drink about half a bottle, stiffen, and then fling the bottle with great fervor. Seems like she settles down after she passes gas or burps."

"What do you do to make these fits go away?" says Zitelli.

"There's nothing much you can do," says the father. "She also keeps her hands in fists. Won't transfer anything. Used to bat a mobile once in a while with her hands, but now she won't even do that anymore."

Zitelli nods ever so curtly as the parents continue to talk about the seizures. They seem like pretty good parents, justifiably concerned. They're young, articulate. They've given some thought to the problem. They explain that four months ago they had taken the child to a gastroenterologist who had tested her for a number of possibilities, including ulcers, but the tests had been negative.

"After listening to your description of these episodes," says Zitelli, "the fact that they are related to eating . . ."

The father interrupts. "You would think she has an ulcer—eats and then gets pain."

"We know that she doesn't have an ulcer. But I think I know what her problem really is," Zitelli continues. "Gastroesophageal reflux."

"Is that serious?" says the mother. "It's serious, isn't it?"

"Don't be ridiculous," the father says. "That's not serious, at least I don't think so. It's heartburn."

"You've got it," says Zitelli.

"I've told my wife frequently that it sounded just like heartburn, but she never listens to what I say."

Zitelli explains to the parents and the intern that a number of tests have to be taken to confirm the diagnosis and, if confirmed, to determine why it is happening. He prescribes a healthy dose of Maalox to provide relief until the tests can be taken and completed. He volunteers to contact Dr. Reynolds "to see how he wants to proceed."

"If she has to stay in the hospital, can I stay with her?" the mother says.

"Absolutely," says Zitelli.

"She's not going to stay by herself," the mother says.

"I understand," says Zitelli, "and, in fact, we might have to give her a Bernstein test." He is referring to a test that makes it possible, in certain gastrointestinal situations, to repeat the symptoms in order for a doctor to observe the problem while it is happening.

The fact that Zitelli has not urged the parents to check the child into Children's or to return to Children's for the necessary tests is related to his function as a pediatricians' pediatrician. He is actually working for Dr. Reynolds as a consultant and can only proceed with the case as far as Reynolds permits. Reynolds is one of about five hundred community-based (private-practice) active staff physicians, who account for about 40 percent of Children's Hospital annual admissions.

Zitelli rushes back to his office to telephone Reynolds and provide a report. During their conversation, Reynolds concurs with Zitelli's diagnosis but decides that the child should be referred back to the original gastroenterologist for the necessary tests.

Zitelli has no choice but to accept Reynolds' decision, but he is disappointed. "The child might be alleviated of her difficulties, the parents might feel better, and the referring doctor might be happy, so that's all to the good," says Zitelli. "But it was my diagnosis, and I guess I wish I could have finished out the case."

Chapter 14

IN 1981, two-year-old Susan Lar-
ris, suffering from incurable liver disease, received a new lease on
life with a then experimental liver transplant, not long after liver
transplant surgeon Thomas Starzl brought his program from the
University of Colorado, where he had been entrenched in research
and experimentation for the past two decades, to Pittsburgh. At the
time, opinion at the University of Pittsburgh and Children's Hospital was divided between those who believed that Starzl's arrival
was a coup—and an equally strong and perhaps more vocal group
who considered it a catastrophe. Not only was liver transplantation
an unproven therapy then, but Starzl's reputation as a cowboy, the
absolute epitome of the surgical personality, magnified the appre-
hensions of the conservative campus.

From nearly the beginning of Starzl's time at Children's, in 1981,
until 1984, when GZMU's relations with the surgeons of the liver
transplant team soured, the group had been intimately involved in
transplantation. They conducted the evaluation of transplant
candidates—an intense physical examination in which the original
diagnosis of the referring physician is confirmed or changed—and
helped with candidate selection and posttransplant care. (GZMU
continues to follow the children they initially guided through the
transplant ordeal, although they do not see new transplant candidates.) Most doctors are unfamiliar with disease affecting the body's
refinery—the liver—so their diagnoses are often incorrect. Even

when the diagnosis is accurate, other avenues of treatment are investigated, for transplantation is the court of last resort, a dangerous surgical intervention with no guarantees of long-range success.

"The worst thing you can do," says pediatric cardiologist Jay Fricker, who conducts the evaluations for the heart transplant program at Children's, "is to transplant someone who doesn't need it, who might have another five or six years until transplantation becomes essential."

It is not the surgery that presents the ultimate challenge, but that indefatigable phenomenon known as "rejection"—meaning that the body's immune system, as a natural and irreversible action, will attempt to reject and destroy foreign objects, including transplanted organs, for an indefinite period of time. A quarter century ago, immunosuppressive medications (medications to suppress or control the immune system) were developed and subsequently refined by Starzl and other surgeon/scientists throughout the world, including azathioprine (trade name Imuran), a chemotherapeutic agent, and steroids (Prednisone). But both drugs were somewhat limited, especially considering the terrible physical and emotional side effects they triggered in most patients, including osteoporosis, diabetes, gout, cataracts, anemia, mood swings, depression, and increased susceptibility to infection.

One of the reasons the University of Pittsburgh was so eager to accommodate Starzl in 1981 was the fact that he had just received permission to conduct experimental clinical trials with a newly developed drug that could potentially unlock the mystery of the immune system without all the destructive side effects caused by the other drugs. Manufactured in Switzerland by Sandoz Pharmaceuticals, and developed by scientist Jean F. Borel, Ph.D., the product, called cyclosporine, had already been tested at Cambridge University in England but had produced disappointingly inconclusive results.

In the Cambridge trials on kidney transplant recipients, cyclosporine did control rejection somewhat more effectively than the formerly developed azathioprine/steroid combination. And even its limited effectiveness came at an unacceptable price, for the drug was not only thought to be nephrotoxic (poisonous to kidneys) but also suspected of inducing lymphoma or lymphoproliferative disease (growth of lymphatic system tumors, usually malignant). But Starzl believed that Cambridge was relying too much on cyclosporine exclusively, while forgetting the advantages of other available immunosuppressives.

In close communication with Borel, Starzl forged ahead, using cyclosporine on his pediatric and adult kidney and liver transplant patients in Pittsburgh in tandem with steroids. This approach not only improved the survival rate of his patients, but by cutting back on the amount of cyclosporine, he was able to alleviate substantially the dangerous side effects of the drug. (The damage that it can do to kidneys has remained a serious although not necessarily insurmountable danger.) In 1983, primarily because of Starzl's work with transplant patients at Pitt, the Food and Drug Administration (FDA) approved cyclosporine for use in all transplant centers on all transplant patients, but only in combination with steroids. Despite the utilization of transplantation to save lives in the past, this event is generally regarded as the leap into the modern age of transplant therapy for which surgeons had long been hoping.

Decreasing the dosage of cyclosporine had controlled the lymphoma problem somewhat, at least in the short run, but not for all patients. About 2 to 3 percent developed malignancies, especially those who had been utilizing this "miracle" immunosuppressive for extended periods of time. Liver transplant recipient Susan Larris had recently returned to Children's with a cancerous tumor adjacent to her kidney. What GZMU would do, how they would proceed, was a question that presented a difficult dilemma. One theory holds that reducing or even withdrawing the cyclosporine will cause the lymphoma to recede and eventually disappear, a strong possibility but with the potential for horrendous consequences for the transplanted liver.

About three months posttransplant, multivisceral recipient Tabatha Foster, with whom Marc Rowe had become so intensely involved, began showing signs, similar to Susan Larris's, of large ulcers or tumors on her liver—indications of lymphoproliferative disease. The tumors went away when cyclosporine was significantly reduced, but the reduction of medication subsequently triggered a second predictable reaction: rejection. Cyclosporine was then increased, inevitably causing the tumor to reappear. A similar scenario might be expected to occur in Susan's situation. "Really, we're shooting from the hip," says Malatack. "Transplantation is a new science, and the lymphoma is one of its newest critical problems."

Originally, lymphoproliferative disease had been attributed to cyclosporine exclusively, but as research into the problem has progressed, scientists have come to believe that it may well be triggered by any sort of immunosuppressive ingested in high dosages over extended periods. Kidney transplant recipients are not nearly as vulnerable, because they take much less immunosuppressive. Long-term immunosuppression is also a threat to heart transplant recipients, causing atherosclerosis, an accumulation of excess plaque in the arteries, in which the reduction of cyclosporine can have little benefit. The only treatment available to these patients is retransplantation. They must repeat the agony of the initial transplant: waiting for an organ, living through surgery, fighting postoperative rejection, and so on.

This is actually Susan Larris's second excursion to Pittsburgh with a problem stemming from the modern age of transplantation. A little more than a year after her first transplant, the little girl's liver went into chronic rejection, meaning that despite the many combinations of immunosuppressives attempted, the immune system was successfully destroying the transplanted liver. To save her from inevitable and painful death, a second transplant was performed. Although Starzl and the pediatricians' pediatricians are in agreement that retransplantation in most cases is an acceptable solution, many medical professionals strongly believe that transplant surgeons go too far, often transplanting three and even four and five organs into dying patients. Starzl's detractors are not necessarily opposed to retransplantation; they just feel that at some point a line must be drawn and the retransplant circuit must be put to a stop.

"I do feel that there is a certain obligation not to abandon patients once a commitment has been made," says Arthur Caplan, director of Bioethics at the University of Minnesota, who conducted a seminar on the subject at Children's Hospital. "At the same time, there is totally inadequate attention to the question 'When will we stop?' "

In justifying his reasoning, Caplan and other bioethicists cite the expense of retransplantation, the decreasing success rate with each transplant because of the ever-weakening condition of the patient, and the fact that each transplant potentially deprives another dying candidate of the possibility of an organ. The latter is especially apropos to a pediatric institution, because there is such a dearth of small donors that nearly half the children with fatal liver and heart disease will die while waiting for a matching organ.

Starzl himself has acknowledged that his "success rate with retransplantation is not as good," while the cost of retransplanting people three times is "prodigious—that's where the $500,000 bills come from, and that's where the terrible suffering and the death occur." But his commitment to the patient to use any conceivable therapy and to fight to the bitter end is inviolable. "If you told physicians who were genuinely concerned with the humanitarian aspects of practice that they could not go forward with the next logical step in care, they would not practice medicine anymore—or they would not comply."

Perhaps the most famous (or infamous) retransplant case is that of seven-year-old Ronnie DeSillers, a saga that took place primarily in Pittsburgh but began in Dade County, Florida, where Ronnie was living with his mother, Maria. Upon learning that Ronnie was dying of liver disease, his elementary school classmates launched a fund-raising drive to collect money enough ($4,000) in order for him to come to Pittsburgh for an evaluation to see if he qualified for a transplant. When the money raised by his classmates was stolen from Ronnie's locker, national attention and compassion were stimulated by newspaper and TV coverage of the theft.

In a nationwide gesture of sympathy and support, money poured in to Maria and Ronnie DeSillers from all over the country, including the White House. President Reagan sent a personal note and a check for $1,000—a gesture that stimulated even more national news. Ronnie's liver transplant, which followed a few weeks later in Pittsburgh, was not successful, however, nor were his second and his third transplant. But each time a transplant occurred, and frequently between transplants, as his condition deteriorated, the media focused attention on Ronnie—and, primarily on a national level, asked the important questions relating to how much or how many transplants are enough, when the line should be drawn. The constant blitz of TV, radio, and print coverage led to a total of approximately $650,000 in donations for Ronnie's treatment, over which his mother automatically became executor.

The dramatic and touching story of the DeSillers saga ended tragically—for everyone concerned. Ronnie died, after suffering months of agony and despair, while awaiting his fourth liver transplant. A few months after his death, Maria DeSillers decided not to pay her balance of approximately $250,000 (about $150,000 had already been paid) to Children's Hospital because she was dissatisfied with the treatment her son had received. For a long time, the hospital, fearing the negative publicity that might result from a protracted battle over the unpaid balance, attempted to collect their money in a quiet way. Maria DeSillers refused to budge, and Children's eventually sued. The case was put in the hands of attorneys for both sides and investigated by Dade County officials, who eventually ordered Maria DeSillers to pay Children's all of the amount owed.

Over a period of many months, Maria DeSillers hurled charges of corporate and medical misconduct at Children's Hospital of Pittsburgh. At different times, she accused the surgeons of transplanting an inferior organ into her son, of giving him a blood transfusion that made him HIV (AIDS) positive, and of mistreating his body after death, knocking it onto the ground. None of the charges were ever substantiated.

At the same time, investigators determined that DeSillers had misdirected donated funds for her own use: rent, automobile, jewelry. She was forced to turn over all the remaining money, less the thousands of dollars that she had already spent, to the state of Florida for distribution to her creditors.

Ronnie DeSillers died after three unsuccessful liver transplants, but it is important to point out that Susan Larris's second transplant had been exceedingly successful, as have a number of retransplantations in children. Over the past five years, she had lived a relatively normal life—at least until now.

"You think you've dodged the bullet," says Malatack, "then you get shot in the back."

Zitelli says, "I went to see the mother and asked her in private how she was doing, but she couldn't get it together to answer. She just broke up."

At this point, says Zitelli, the parents are withholding any concrete information from Susan about her condition—a tactic GZMU and most other pediatricians do not endorse, because at nine years old children usually have a fairly decent understanding of the life-and-death issues surrounding them.

At the very least, says Malatack, Susan must have very strong suspicions about what is happening. "I'm sure she knows that this is something much more serious than anything else that has ever occurred in her course of treatment. She's back here, for starters; she's in the hospital. And they are eliminating cyclosporine. The surgeons have told her repeatedly in the past, 'Do not ever miss this dose of cyclosporine,' and then she comes in here and they stop it cold. That's got to be pretty confusing to a kid.

"What happens when we try to hide certain things from children, is that the kids often end up faking their ignorance to try to appease their parents. They feel that's what they're expected to do." He admits that the parents have the right to determine how the child is approached, and the doctor is obliged to work in the manner in which they are directed. "You try to let them understand that this is not the right way to handle things from a psychosocial standpoint. But that's all you can do."

Chapter 15

ZITELLI'S next appointment that afternoon is another liver transplant recipient, Alan Sollenberger, who received his first organ in March 1986 and his second in May of the same year. Alan, seven years old, is walking very stiffly as he enters Zitelli's office. Big red splotches have recently appeared all over his body, his mother reports, and his feet were swelled up "like sausages. And they're burning," says the mother, "because of the high levels of cyclosporine in his body."

Mrs. Sollenberger is guessing, but as a veteran of three years of coping with an array of problems stemming from liver transplantation and the necessary onslaught of immunosuppression, she is much more knowledgeable about the practical aspects of life after transplantation and the use of immunosuppressive medications than the average pediatrician. She is probably right about the cyclosporine.

One of the more troublesome aspects in the treatment of transplant recipients is the maintenance of an adequate balance of whatever immunosuppressive regimen—cyclosporine, Prednisone, and, in some cases, azathioprine—the patient might be taking. There are, unfortunately, no standard formulas; Alan Sollenberger, Susan Larris, and every other transplant recipient will require different amounts of each immunosuppressive to stave off rejection, with the proper balance determined by the surgeons through a long trial-and-error process, frequently requiring months of juggling.

Despite the precision with which the formula can be fine-tuned, side effects inevitably occur. When they do, the surgeons prescribe additional medications—insulin for the diabetes caused by the steroids; Lasix (furosemide), a diuretic, to relieve fluid retention. Often, the addition of these side-effect-countering medications into the bloodstream will disrupt cyclosporine levels, resulting in one of the two extremes the doctors are trying to avoid. Although Alan Sollenberger has not yet reached either extreme, he is clearly a victim of the side-effect-countering drugs.

Zitelli seats the Sollenbergers side by side in his office, with Alan in a chair between them. Mr. Sollenberger, a dairy farmer from central Pennsylvania, is tall and robust with a round face, broad shoulders, a large stomach, and ample ears, an image that is enhanced by his crewcut. Mrs. Sollenberger is also robust and energetic-looking, as are Alan's two siblings, whose photos she carries in her wallet. In stark contrast, Alan is pale and lethargic, with cherubic cheeks and an overall puffiness—distortions caused by the Prednisone. His arms and face are also inordinately hairy for a child of seven—a side effect of the cyclosporine.

Zitelli begins by explaining that Alan is immunosuppressed, so he is more susceptible to colds—dangerous to most transplant recipients because such minor infections can lead to pneumonia, more serious infections, and death. Alan's susceptibility is complicated by the fact that he is allergic to penicillin and other antibiotics. Over a period of time, however, doctors have discovered that his system can process one antibiotic, erythromycin (trade name Erythrocin), which will effectively fight off infection. A consequence of erythromycin, however, is that it inhibits Alan's ability to process cyclosporine, which, in turn, leads to higher amounts of cyclosporine in the body, causing swelling, lethargy, and other problems.

"When his legs started to hurt, his sleeping was affected," said Mrs. Sollenberger. "Now he gets up at night and sleeps during the day. He eats, but I have to carry him to the table. He's getting sicker and weaker all the time."

"Not too long ago," said the father, "he was filled out and healthy. Fighting with his big brothers and rolling around on the ground. Then he got sick, and then he got sick again and again. He lost weight and muscle. Now he's definitely gone backward."

The mother asks, "Do you think his resistance is so low that we should keep him out of school? That's what our pediatrician at home thinks."

"No," says Zitelli. "Most of the germs that he could get at school are viral, and for those problems erythromycin is not needed."

"I'm confused." Mrs. Sollenberger shakes her head.

"We've gotten into a vicious cycle," says Zitelli. "The erythromycin wreaks havoc with his cyclosporine levels, and when the level gets high, it makes him more susceptible to infection, which causes even more need for erythromycin. The solution is to get him off erythromycin and to find another antibiotic to treat his infections."

The mother momentarily changes the subject. "Alan is really getting to be smart. When he can't get to school, we have a teacher, a newcomer to the area, originally from the city, who comes to the house. She was showing him a picture one day. She said, 'What is this, Alan?'

"And he said, 'Guernsey.'

"And she said, 'Alan, come on. You know what this is.'

"And he said, 'Guernsey.'

" 'Alan,' she said, 'this is a milking cow.'

" 'I know it's a milking cow,' he answered, 'a special milking cow called a Guernsey.' "

Zitelli chuckles as he escorts the Sollenbergers back to the examination room. "Does it hurt him to put shoes on him?" he asks.

"Can you ever get them off?" the mother says. "His feet are purple."

As Alan's vital signs are taken, Zitelli explains to me that he was influential in persuading the family to proceed with a liver transplant in 1986. The Sollenbergers are very typical country people, with old-fashioned values, essentially isolated from the world of high-technology medicine. Transplantation was foreign to the parents, especially the father, who worried whether he could afford it. The farm was barely making it. Could he handle the burden of a chronically ill child, along with $5,000 to $10,000 of medication every year? Mr. Sollenberger finally agreed to the transplant with tears in his eyes. Two months later, retransplantation was necessary, and there was another long and involved decision. Luckily, it turned out well.

Like most other pediatric patients who traveled the long road through transplantation, Alan was unable to start school with children of his age. Consequently, when recently evaluated for school placement, he tested in the retarded range. But Zitelli says that once pediatric liver transplant recipients get back into a normal rhythm of life, they advance quickly, and in time they catch up with peers. Zitelli is the author of the in-depth and up-to-date study, "Changes in Life-Style After Liver Transplantation," of sixty-five pediatric recipients regularly observed for up to five years. (Ninety were transplanted during that period; 72 percent were alive at the time the study was conducted.)

According to Zitelli, more than three-quarters of the patients were currently either in age-appropriate school grades or one year behind. The most common reason for delay was chronic illness prior to transplantation. Motor skill was significantly improved after transplantation. "It was not uncommon for parents to report, 'He runs, plays tag, climbs up and down trees, plays Frisbee and ball, and swings on swings. He couldn't do any of that before,'" says Zitelli. Generally, the behavior of the patient and the siblings also improved after transplantation. Children were more spontaneous and cooperative. Parents also tended to view themselves as more relaxed.

"Despite overall improvement, parents still did not perceive their child's behavior as entirely normal, however: behavioral immaturity tended to persist after transplantation; defiance and aggression sometimes were seen; fear of infection and medication side effects remained." Zitelli also noted in his study that parents continued to express numerous fears, not only of rejection and the side effects of medication, but also of medical expenses, as in the case of Mr. Sollenberger. Parents also tended to be overprotective, as evidenced by Mrs. Sollenberger's reluctance to send Alan back to school.

"I know it makes you feel vulnerable," Zitelli told her. "But we believe we should put children back into the mainstream as soon as possible."

The mother nods but is obviously unconvinced. "If you say so," she says, "but . . ."

"Alan, can you blow this light out?" Zitelli proceeds with his examination, switching on the little flashlight he will use to look into Alan's ears.

Alan keeps staring straight ahead, as if in a trance. He seems even more pale and fragile without his clothes on; there is a large crescent-shaped scar across his abdominal area.

"He doesn't want to play," Zitelli says. "He's probably sorry he didn't bring that terrible snake. The worst kind. A black rubber snake, about a foot long."

"But the snake broke," says Mr. Sollenberger. "You bet we fixed it up, though. It's as good as new."

"Did you have Dr. Starzl do the surgery on the snake?" asked Zitelli.

"No, it was taped."

"I hate that snake," Zitelli says to Alan, who looks silently and impassively back at him.

"When Alan is feeling better, he's usually got a few more things to say," Mr. Sollenberger observes. "Especially about that there snake. He'd be holding it up and scaring Dr. Zitelli to death."

Alan's legs are thin and spindly, and his chest is sunken, especially compared with his protruding stomach. "Was his liver bigger than it should have been?" Mrs. Sollenberger asks.

"I don't know," says Zitelli, "but I doubt it."

"I thought they mentioned that his liver was a little bigger at the time of the surgery," said the mother.

Zitelli begins to squeeze Alan's feet, then he puts his hand on Alan's leg and with two fingers raps down hard over the back of his hand, making a sound like a knocking door. Alan's cries are loud and piercing, but Zitelli continues undaunted. "Get him dressed. I'm going to arrange to get him an abdominal sonogram."

"Alan doesn't look well," Zitelli tells me as we return to his office. "He's pale, washed-out, and his skin isn't taut." As to what these symptoms indicate, Zitelli says, "I don't know, but they worry me."

What about Mrs. Sollenberger's concern that the liver might be too large? "The liver couldn't be too large or they wouldn't have been able to close him up. But his spleen is massive, swelled, and I would like to know why."

"Do you have any questions?" Zitelli asks when the parents return to the office with Alan, now dressed.

"No," says the father.

Zitelli laughs and points accusingly at Mr. Sollenberger. "Yes, you do. I know you. You're going to go home and ask your wife, as usual, all the things you didn't want to ask me, and she's not going to have all the answers you want, so she'll have to call me up and ask me."

The parents do ask a couple of follow-up questions, but in fact Zitelli cannot really provide too many answers until he receives the results of the sonogram. He promises to be in touch as soon as possible.

"One more thing, Alan," Zitelli says as the Sollenbergers depart, "whatever you do, when you come back here next time"—he pauses to shake his finger at the little boy—"I'm warning you, now, don't you dare bring that snake."

In December 1987, a study similar to Zitelli's, written by pediatric cardiologist Jay Fricker and nurse specialist Kathy Lawrence, was published in the *Journal of Heart Transplantation*. It focused on the heart transplant patients at Children's Hospital over a three-year period. The study, although involving much smaller numbers of patients (twelve), is quite representative of both the positives and the negatives of organ transplantation—and the vital questions that remain unanswered.

"Interviews with parents revealed incredible changes in the child's routine before and after transplantation," Lawrence and Fricker note. "Before surgery, all children were homebound, and most needed frequent hospitalizations. No child was able to do self-care without assistance or participate regularly in tutoring sessions. No one had an age-appropriate friend. Interest in play or other interaction with the environment was almost nonexistent. Most of the child's concern was toward his body. In each case, the illness of the child virtually curtailed family outings. One mother graphically told of never being able to take her wheelchair-bound, diuretic-dependent child outside the home. There simply were not enough handicapped bathroom facilities. It was even difficult for his mother to leave home with the rest of the family because baby-sitters were afraid to stay with this ill-looking child.

"Postoperatively, the story changed for these children. All were ambulatory, competent in self-care, and able to attend school regularly. Grades had not declined from those achieved before the onset of severe illness. Six had at least one age-appropriate friend and engaged in age-appropriate play. Only two children needed to return to the hospital for periods longer than one week. All families were able to enjoy outings together once again."

Potentially, organ transplantation can be incredibly positive therapy, but the end results are very unpredictable and inconsistent. In the Lawrence-Fricker study, three of the twelve recipients died soon after surgery, while two more recipients died within eight months after transplantation; two additional recipients died after the study was published. Considering the cost ($100,000 to $200,000) and the open-ended questions about the future of the survivors, many transplant professionals, including Fricker, doubt the value of transplantation as long-term therapy, especially for children. Fricker points out that nationally, only 30 percent of all transplant recipients are alive a decade after surgery; in five years a recipient has an even chance of surviving.

"In an adult, say a forty-year-old man who lives to be forty-five, that's significant, in terms of his family, helping his children to develop and mature. When it comes to children, I'm not sure transplantation is the right thing to do, considering that there's a fifty-fifty chance that a three- or four-year-old will live only to age eight or nine. So who are you doing the transplant for," Fricker wonders, "the kid or his parents?"

Jeffrey Malatack voiced a similar question the day that doctors had given up on Susan Larris and sent her home, ostensibly to die. "It's easy to see the benefits of organ transplantation when dealing with adults," Malatack told me. "But it's a completely different matter when you help two-year-olds who really had no concept of life to begin with to extend their lives up until nine—and then they die. You begin to question what you're doing."

Chapter 16

I AM sitting in the playroom, watching as Judy Cochran of Birmingham, Alabama, and Rashad, a little Arab boy, the recent recipient of a liver transplant, blow bubbles at one another. Rashad is attached to an intravenous unit, like a puppy on a leash. He can't go far, but he covers his ground with nervous quickness. Off in the corner is another little boy, huddled with one of the hospital maintenance people, building a truck with a plastic Erector Set.

My eyes are fixed on Judy's daughter, Kellie, whose legs and arms are like twigs but whose blue eyes shine with a kind of detached fascination. Instinctively she reaches out to embrace the bubbles, which lazily evade her tiny and awkward grasp.

The nurse comes in with Kellie's many medicines, loaded in narrow dispensers, and injects them one by one into her mouth. Kellie accepts each injection with a glazed-over kind of annoyance. Medicine is nothing new for this little girl; medicine is something she has tolerated from the very beginning of her short and painful life.

A shot of pink drool suddenly spills from Kellie's mouth and rolls down her T-shirt. It is only noon, but this is the third outfit Kellie has ruined. "Well, Kellie," Judy says, "the next time you'll be back to the hospital gown."

Kellie is crying as Judy undresses her, but this is what the little girl has wanted all along. Kellie's symptoms are not as pronounced as some of the other patients suffering from liver disease whom I have seen, but they are extraordinarily severe nonetheless. She has the brownish-yellow cast—jaundice—and the bloated belly caused by the buildup of poisonous fluid and ammonia. Her arms and legs are next to nothing in size; my forefinger is nearly as wide as her wrist.

Kellie is two years old. For more than a year she has weighed fifteen pounds, although it is obvious by the look of her that she is being well cared for. A lot of people have gone out of their way to make life tolerable for the little girl, but with her emaciated frame I can't help thinking of the pictures I have seen of concentration camp victims. For the past month, she has been waiting in Pittsburgh for organs to materialize so that she can be transplanted. Her life is in imminent jeopardy.

When her clothes come off, Kellie quiets down, and when Judy takes out the hairbrush, Kellie's eyes brighten slightly. "This," says Judy, "is Kellie's favorite toy."

Judy rubs the hairbrush over Kellie's little body, and for the first time I see more than simple signs of acceptance in Kellie's wondrous blue eyes. She is not capable of much emotion, but there is a flicker of relief that seems to make her look like any other normal two-year-old, at least momentarily. The incessant itching caused by liver disease is the greatest torment; adult patients I have interviewed describe this itching as so unrelenting that it seems to emanate from the inside out. Kellie is not strong enough to put up much of a struggle, but when Judy attempts to dress her, Kellie begins to squirm and cry. "Kellie, you can't stay undressed," Judy says. "I keep this up, I'll scratch your skin away."

She pauses to caress Kellie with the brush once more, and then to apply some lotion to the little girl's arms and feet and hands, but every time she tries to put on the little shirt and overalls, Kellie screams louder. Judy is steadfast. "Kellie has a mind of her own, but so do I."

It is a slow process, but Judy knows what she is doing. If Kellie will only give an inch, will allow her shirt to be slipped over her head, then Judy will scratch, so that Kellie will relax, and Judy can gain more headway. A sleeve, a leg, a button. In a while, Kellie is dressed.

We put Kellie in a stroller and head down to the cafeteria. We sit, talk, Judy smoking a cigarette, Kellie sipping from a straw in a can of Mountain Dew. Judy says that the last time they came to the cafeteria, Kellie vomited a day's worth of food at the first sip of Coke. Mountain Dew seems to be easier on her stomach. "Kellie's always vomiting, but she can usually keep down a little bit more than she coughs up."

Judy's life here seems to be simple enough—and terrible. She changes Kellie's clothes four or five times a day, then goes home at night to the Ronald McDonald House, where she and many other families are located while children and siblings are bedbound at Children's Hospital, to do Kellie's laundry and snatch a couple of hours of sleep. She talks to the nurses and tries to feed Kellie, begging and pleading with her to eat. At a restaurant recently, while on a hospital pass, Judy discovered that Kellie loved ketchup, so now all her food is soaked with ketchup—anything to help increase caloric intake and enhance her failing strength. One day she has hashbrowns with ketchup at lunch, and then bites of barbecued chicken for dinner.

Before and after feeding, there is always bathing, and then oil applied to her skin every few hours. Kellie's "bum" is nonexistent; skin sags from the narrow trunk of bone. And between everything, there is scratching with the hairbrush, forever scratching. Kellie also scratches on her own, digging desperately into her nose and ears, raking her tiny fingers through her scalp, and picking at her feet.

Two or three dozen times a day, Judy fits Kellie into the portable stroller and wheels her around and around the long corridors of the hospital. "We cover miles this way; my legs are in great shape," says Judy. "People tell me that there are many stages to live through during the transplant process, but this waiting, watching while my daughter is dying, is worse than anything I've ever imagined."

Judy and I are in the cafeteria for only a few minutes when the Mountain Dew starts coming up all over Kellie's fresh clothes. I collect a couple of napkins, but Kellie is soaked, and Judy decides to take her back up to the floor. I will carry the stroller later.

By the time I get upstairs, Kellie is screaming. Four or five other babies on the floor are screaming, too. Watching an adult suffer and die from liver and/or heart disease is difficult enough, but this is too much, almost surreal in its cruel and uncontrollable intensity. Children are so helpless, unable to communicate their problems, unable to raise the roof with indignation with their complaints, yet so extraordinarily courageous and trusting in their innocence. It's this courage and trust that touch your heart. Unblinkingly, they give themselves over to the adult world, frightened, pained, and confused, and we, who have not yet been able to solve the simple problem of bringing nutrition and basic health care to all people in need, are expected to unravel the mysteries of a tiny human body—the most complicated machine on earth.

I tell Judy I have to go, I have an appointment, I'll see her later. I walk out into the corridor, stop, and turn around. "Is there anything I can get you?"

As usual, she is smiling, but her smile is now just a tight and twitching line across her pale and desperate face. "A little bit of sanity," she says.

I stare at her helplessly, drawing my shoulders up tightly against my neck in a slow and nervous shrug.

"Is that too much to ask?"

"No," I said, "I guess not."

In order for a liver or heart transplant to occur, the recipient must be matched to a brain-dead donor in a number of critical ways, including height, weight, and blood type. Size is one of the main reasons so many children die—perhaps 50 percent of all infants with heart or liver disease—while waiting for an organ. Not many small children are involved in suicides or auto accidents—the diseaseless deaths, usually neurological in origin, that produce organs for transplant.

As children grow older, the parameters become more flexible. An organ from a thirty-pound child would be too big to fit into an infant, for example, but a liver or heart of a small adult would function effectively in a child who weighs sixty to seventy pounds. Blood types must remain consistent in heart transplants, but in certain critical situations, liver transplant surgeons will cross blood types. Or when blood type matches and size doesn't, they will resect a liver (cut off a piece) in an attempt to save a life when no other options are available. Age, race, and sex of either donor or recipient have no bearing, and once a heart, liver, or kidney is transplanted from one child to another, the organ will grow in tandem with the rest of the body.

With some exceptions and complications (tissue typing), similar parameters exist for matching and transplanting kidneys. A primary difference between kidney and extrarenal (other than kidney) transplants is that a human being, although endowed with two kidneys, can live a healthy life with one kidney and, under certain circumstances, give the other to a spouse, sibling, or friend suffering from kidney disease. Living-related transplants were established more than a decade before cadaveric (from a brain-dead donor) transplants were made viable. The first successful homograft, or human-to-human transplant, occurred in 1954 in Boston at Peter Bent Brigham Hospital. The donor and the recipient were identical twins and thus perfectly matched—so much so that the recipient lived a healthy life for three years before dying of infections unrelated to the transplant. Surgeons have been pushing at the ever-increasing boundaries between life and death since that first transplant thirty-five years ago. Today, one of the newest frontiers is bone marrow transplantation.

Jeffrey Malatack, who recently completed a six-month fellowship in bone marrow transplantation at the University of Pennsylvania while on sabbatical from Pittsburgh, says that bone marrow transplantation—the act of injecting marrow from one human being into another—does not require the same diligence, experience, and sophisticated surgical skill necessary for organ transplantation. He says, "You can teach a chimp to do it in a week."

The skill in bone marrow transplantation comes in the management of the patient after transplantation until the transplanted bone marrow becomes a fully functioning and interactive part of the body. This is not dissimilar to the postoperative challenges facing organ transplant surgeons, but because bone marrow transplantation is a newer and perhaps more delicate science, the day-to-day decisions are often more crucial—especially regarding immunosuppression and the lifelong threat of rejection. Jeff Malatack and I are heading for one of the Children's Hospital oncology units to see a bone marrow recipient, Clinton Szemanski, who was transplanted two months ago. Whereas in organ transplantation "rejection" refers to the reaction of the body's immune system against the transplanted organ, Malatack tells me, bone marrow transplanters fear the exact opposite reaction—graft-versus-host disease, in which the transplanted marrow refuses to accept the body into which it has been injected.

Before entering Clinton's room, we stop in a small anteroom to wash our hands and mask our faces. Malatack explains that the room is cleaned daily with an antibacterial agent, and he describes the ventilation system as a "positive-pressure environment," meaning that the air pressure in the room is higher than in the anteroom, which is higher than the air pressure in the corridor, so that germs or viruses in either the anteroom or corridor will not be carried by draft into Clinton's room. Because of the threat of rejection, all transplant recipients are immunosuppressed, but bone marrow recipients are even more vulnerable to rejection and infection. Before the transplant, they are injected with a heavy dose of chemotherapy to eradicate the disease and the affected marrow. It is at that point—at their weakest and most vulnerable—that the life saving marrow is injected into the bloodstream. "It works just like a blood transfusion. Just put it in a vein; it finds its own way home. We call this the 'good earth' theory. Blood cells kind of sense where they belong."

He says that there is a patient in the hospital now whose own marrow was frozen in advance. "This is a girl who had leukemia but was in remission. At that point, we salvaged marrow as a safeguard if and when the cancer returned, which is exactly what happened."

Malatack performed a number of transplants as a fellow at Children's of Philadelphia, where doctors would thaw the entire batch of marrow, frozen in a large plastic bag, and then rush it from the lab to the patient. When he returned to Pittsburgh, he learned that Montefiore Hospital, another university-affiliated hospital with a large adult bone marrow transplant program, was freezing the marrow in small bags—25 cc per bag—and thawing each bag as needed, in the room. Not only is this easier, but if patients happen to have a bad reaction to the marrow for any reason, the entire batch, which cannot be refrozen, won't be ruined. The marrow is frozen in a substance called DMSO, a solvent used to facilitate absorption of medicines through the skin, which contains a strong garlic odor, and for a day or two afterward, the patient will be emanating a garlic aura.

Malatack says that within a month, enough marrow will be making new blood cells so that patients' radical isolation can be ended. "But generally, it is going to take at least six months until the marrow is doing all the things it should be doing and you can start being around people again without being fearful of infection." Only one of each four children provided with a bone marrow transplant will be cured.

Malatack distinguishes between whole organ transplantation and bone marrow transplantation in one significant way: the possibility in livers and hearts to change the organs if rejection or infection is discovered to be irreversible. "In liver transplantation, you try to get the immune system to accept a foreign organ, but what you are doing in bone marrow transplantation is changing the immune system. The only way to do that is by destroying the immune system with superlethal doses of chemotherapy. You give those superlethal doses of chemotherapy a second time, you're much more likely to kill the patient from the toxic effects of the drugs. So it's much different in approach."

Clinton, four years old, is suffering from Sanfilippo syndrome, which essentially means that a special and important enzyme is missing from his body, including his marrow. "It's a progressive disease," says Malatack, "and had he not had a transplant, he would have become progressively less functional neurologically" and died in a vegetative state within the next six years.

Marrow from siblings is much more likely to match than marrow from parent to child. "The father and the mother conceive the child, and so usually you will find that the child's marrow only partially matches each of his or her parents." When tests were performed to determine if Clinton's younger brother would be a satisfactory match for Clinton, Malatack discovered that the sibling also suffered from Sanfilippo syndrome. The father, however, turned out to be an acceptable match for Clinton, an unusual circumstance, but neither parent could help the younger son. Malatack then proceeded with Clinton's transplant, while sending the brother's matching requirements to the national bone marrow registry. "Our hope is that there's someone, somewhere in this world, who has registered his or her matching marrow and who is willing to come to Pittsburgh to save this kid's life."

In addition to the medical problems haunting both Szemanski children, the family was confronted with a disorienting and frustrating complication: the insurance company decided not to pay for Clinton's procedure (approximately $50,000) because bone marrow transplantation was, at that time, "experimental." But as long as the Szemanskis were local residents, Malatack could proceed with the transplant, knowing that payment was guaranteed through the Children's Hospital's Free Care Fund. Now, on top of their other problems, the family was in arbitration with the insurance company in an attempt to force a reversal of decision. The Free Care Fund would make up the difference between the actual charges and whatever the Szemanskis could afford to pay, while the Szemanskis were attempting to force the company to assume the entire bill for both children.

As we enter the room, Clinton displays what Malatack calls a "gargoyle syndrome," a puffiness throughout the entire body, noticeable especially in his cheeks, caused by the Prednisone (steroids), one of his primary immunosuppressive medications. Clinton had been discharged about three weeks ago after a two-month in-hospital siege, but Malatack had recently readmitted him because the child was experiencing difficulty in breathing and in holding down his food. At the same time, a rash of unknown origin had appeared in patches over most of his body. Because bone marrow transplantation is, in fact, experimental, it is standard practice to readmit patients for observation and treatment whenever inexplicable complications of any kind occur.

"This is such a voodoo kind of therapy," Malatack adds, "you can never tell what might happen. He could lose his graft; he could get any kind of infection imaginable, he's so terribly immunosuppressed. In addition to GVH (graft-versus-host), there is an entity associated with bone marrow transplantation called 'bone marrow transplant pneumonia'; it has a very high mortality—eighty percent of those patients usually die within a few weeks of when they get it." There are an equal number of patients who get clinical pneumonia, along with numerous other viral infections such as cytomegalo virus, which kills more posttransplant patients than any other single entity other than rejection.

There is a tiny mirror in a yellow plastic frame attached to Clinton's crib, and periodically Malatack directs and redirects Clinton's attention to the face—Clinton's face—reflecting back at him. Malatack is a very gentle practitioner who has a way of conducting a thorough examination or a complicated conversation in an extraordinarily underwhelming manner. Described by his partners and other colleagues as "the idealist," "the ethicist," the man most "left-of-center" of the group, Malatack gives the impression of being kind of dour, unsmiling, and overburdened in a worldly sort of way. But his concerns are quite compassionate, especially when the extent to which health care can be offered must be measured by parameters of dollars rather than need. The Guatemalan child has been on his mind since the initial diagnosis, and as we walked through the hospital that morning he made repeated references to the inequitable division of resources—even in his own area.

"We can give bone marrow transplants for $50,000 because a certain child lives in western Pennsylvania and qualifies for the Free

Care Fund or has the right insurance coverage, but we can't fix this kid's heart because he lives in another country. The nurses are here, the doctors are here, the facilities are available; it's not like we're snowed under with patients at this particular moment. So why can't we just do this procedure and help this child?" he asks rhetorically. Then he answers his question with a grimace and a shrug. "Because it costs $50,000."

Malatack has written a letter to the medical director of the hospital, William Donaldson, who could authorize the surgery for reasons of compassion. The little boy's foster mother has vowed that she would adopt the child and move him permanently to Pittsburgh to avail herself of the Free Care Fund if there is no other way.

As he gently lifts Clinton's diaper and follows the line of a red-dotted rash that spreads up and down his trunk to the palms of his hands and the bottoms of his feet, Malatack explains that graft-versus-host disease primarily affects the skin, the liver, and the GI tract. "You look for nasal flaring to assess the respiratory effort, and you look at the progression of the rash. You also look for jaundice—an indication that he is developing liver problems. People who get GVH that includes the GI tract and the skin but doesn't affect the liver have a better prognosis."

At the completion of the examination, Malatack turns to the father, a large pie-faced man with an easy and open grin. The mother stayed home last night to care for Clinton's brother. "How ya doin?" Malatack says.

"Pretty good. Clinton got eleven and a half hours' sleep last night, so he's doing pretty well, also. I mean, his breathing seems slow compared to yesterday—at least to me. He had a banana and some ice cubes for breakfast, the first food he's eaten and kept down in days."

"His rash looks better," Malatack says, "but we'll leave him on the IV [because of the danger to his GI tract] for a couple of days, and then, if everything looks all right, we'll switch him back to oral medications."

They talk for a little while longer, and as Malatack is ready to leave the father says, "Who you gonna take Sunday?" He is referring to the upcoming Steeler game.

Malatack says he's going to take the 'Skins, and seven points.

"Forget it," says the father. "I'm only betting even money."

"Not with me," Malatack says.

Malatack is laughing and shaking his head as we leave the room. "Clinton was admitted over the weekend with the rash and GI infection. It was actually the kid's darkest moment since the transplant, but on Monday morning the father told me, 'I think he's going to make it. I feel confident.' "

"Why?" Malatack had asked. This was obviously not the ideal time to feel confident.

" 'Well,' says the father, 'because the Steelers won on Sunday.' "

Chapter 17

A FEW days after Susan Larris died, I spent an afternoon with Basil Zitelli at the Continuity Clinic, which takes place each weekday afternoon at Children's Hospital so that residents can see patients—the same patients throughout their three-year residency—on a regular basis. Zitelli serves as preceptor, as do Bruce Rosenthal and his colleagues in the ER, providing information and answers for those young doctors who need help, while periodically observing and subsequently evaluating each resident's overall performance. Zitelli and the other preceptors will prepare regular written evaluations and meet with each resident to discuss their weaknesses and strengths as doctors and communicators.

Whereas the Walk-In Clinic is part of the Emergency Room and deals in "episodic" care, the Continuity Clinic is a rare "longitudinal" experience; the resident through his or her rotations will normally not have the opportunity to establish and sustain a long-term relationship with a patient and family, an experience that much more closely represents private-practice pediatrics than most of the situations they'll confront in the hospital. Zitelli says that 50 percent of the residents at Children's in Pittsburgh will go immediately into private practice, in contrast to the more esoteric programs, such as at Boston Children's (Harvard), where "if you don't go into academia, people think there's something wrong with you."

Molly O'Gorman and Laurie Penix were both to choose academic careers. Penix received a fellowship in infectious disease at the

University of Washington in Seattle, while O'Gorman will pursue her studies in gastroenterology at Johns Hopkins, a position she captured with the support of Zitelli, a well-respected alumnus of the institution. When I first met O'Gorman and Penix, they were halfway through their three-year residency, having put behind them the difficult internship, or first-year residency period—the most crushing because of the demands of time (an intern will often go thirty-six hours without sleep) and because of the transition from being taught and guided in medical school to actually performing the various high-pressure duties of a doctor on real patients.

The second year of residency was the most exciting and consuming, both residents agreed, because you were thrown into a series of new and demanding situations once every four to six weeks but had a certain amount of experience and confidence to buttress your newness. The third year was most enjoyable because the resident could choose from a number of electives—cardiology, infectious disease, otolaryngology, for instance—and the hours were not so demanding. There was time to do some of your own research in the laboratory and to take charge of less experienced interns and residents, helping them make decisions without having to consult an attending physician whenever problems occurred. The responsibility the resident or "house officer" is afforded fulfills a wish and a goal that was established early in life. "I was born and bred to be a physician," Laurie Penix once told me. "It was as clear as day from the first grade onward that I would someday be a doctor."

O'Gorman's father, a prominent surgeon in Buffalo, New York, instilled the spirit of medicine in her from a very early age. The O'Gormans lived on a sprawling and beautiful farm in the country, and she remembers that there were ten phones on the property so that the hospital could reach her father at a moment's notice. Ironically, although her grades were high enough, she tested poorly and was unable to get into a good medical school after college. So she pursued a master's degree in science, then went to work at the highly regarded Great Ormond Street Hospital in London for six months before heading back to America, where she assisted a surgeon, whom she calls "Dr. Joe," at a clinic in rural Alaska. She then reapplied for medical school and was accepted at the State University of New York at Buffalo.

Most people discuss the difficult demands of residency; many books, articles, and films have captured the exhausting schedule and constant pressure. What I noticed more than anything, though, was how the experience, the day-to-day clash with life's realities, had aged and changed Penix and O'Gorman and the other residents I came to know. Here were two young women from the upper middle class, who had lived an essentially protected and carefully monitored life for their first twenty-three or twenty-four years, suddenly thrust into the violence, the blood, the poverty, the tragedy that a high-acuity hospital—even a children's hospital—in a major metropolitan area regularly attracts.

I got to know O'Gorman as a friend outside of the hospital rather well because we share similar athletic interests—running long distances and working out regularly at a nearby club. Although O'Gorman was not particularly expressive, the ravages of the day appeared on her face in the evenings, especially after 12 hours in the ER, on transport duty, or in the ICU. So often, her face would look puffy from sleepiness and pasty from being indoors for so long; exercise buoyed her spirits and brought color back to her cheeks. "Bad day?" I would say to her, sooner or later.

"Don't ask," she'd answer, rolling her eyes, pushing her short blond hair back behind her ears. "It's not worth talking about; I just want it to go away."

Penix told me that the biggest shock of her residency was "coming across families—parents and kids—that I didn't like. I never thought that would happen because I have always loved people and gotten along with them so well." With pessimistic irony, she had formulated in her mind what she chose to call "a Pythagorean theorem of pediatrics," defined as, "the nicer the kid or the family, the more horrible the disease the kid has. It just seems to correlate." Families who are always "cussing and calling you filthy names in the ER survive amazing insults and never seem to have chronic problems. The nicer the family is, however, the worse the complications."

Although Penix's comments are overstated, it is probably true that all health-care professionals—doctors, nurses, technicians, even veterans like Basil Zitelli—suffer to a certain extent from Penix's "Pythagorean theorem of pediatrics," especially at particularly difficult points in their lives as physicians.

Zitelli seemed reflective and low-key the day we spent at the Continuity Clinic, somewhat depressed. Not much was going on, so he had time to reflect and ponder Susan Larris's death—which, although not unexpected, came as a blow nonetheless, a fact of life that he could not easily hide. Zitelli is blessed with a distinctly honest face and a flat and straightforward manner, a man unaccustomed to deception. Talking about Susan Larris was clearly uncomfortable for him, but he seemed bent upon doing it—in fact, he seemed to need to talk. I was willing to move on to other subjects, but Zitelli continued to turn the conversation back to Susan Larris and other long-term pediatric transplant recipients.

"Many children are coming back, three or four or five years now, posttransplant. A few are testing HIV [AIDS] positive because of the blood they received in transfusion in the early eighties, but now that the blood is being so carefully screened, AIDS won't be a problem in the future. And that wasn't the fault of transplantation anyway. Many kids are also returning for biliary [bile duct] reconstruction, but although this is a difficult surgery, it is fixable." But the children returning to the scene of their transplant with lymphoproliferative disease represent a potentially disastrous problem that is caused by the transplant itself—which was initially the one and only therapy available to save their lives. "Susan Larris's death," says Zitelli, "quite honestly shakes the foundation of my faith."

Zitelli's faith may well have been further tested when, a few days later, Alan Sollenberger was rushed to the Children's Hospital ICU with pneumonia, a side effect of high-dosage cyclosporine therapy. Alan was experiencing difficulty in breathing and was ventilated (had a breathing tube inserted in his windpipe). Lymphoproliferative disease was suspected and later confirmed.

For the first few weeks, I steered clear of the Sollenbergers, hoping that Alan would get better so that he would be transferred to a private room, where I could more comfortably visit. But Alan's condition further deteriorated to the point where the discomfort, the swelling and burning from the ventilator—he was "tubed" through his nose—was becoming intolerable to him. Not only could he not communicate, but the pain was so great that he was expending every ounce of his waning strength attempting to rip the ventilator off his face, an effort causing further swelling and pain.

The day I visit, Mrs. Sollenberger is home with Alan's two older brothers for the first time in three weeks, and Mr. Sollenberger has come in to watch over his ailing son, who is making very slow but positive progress. Here is a man obviously at home in the backwoods on his farm, the same land tilled by his father and his father's father, but generally unhappy and uncomfortable in a city atmosphere— especially in the frantic life-and-death world of an ICU of a pediatric hospital. But Alan's father eases his large frame into the wooden rocker placed carefully beside his son's bed, and with his red face frozen in a friendly, welcoming, country-style smile, begins rocking rhythmically. I sit beside him and for a while we rock together, until one of the ICU doctors approaches, asking for consent to surgically insert a tracheostomy into Alan's throat so that the tube in his nose can be removed.

Although Alan has had a tracheostomy once before and it was a simple and minor invasive procedure, and although Mr. Sollenberger clearly understands that the trach would considerably ease Alan's discomfort, he suddenly finds himself unable to make what seems to everyone else to be an incredibly easy decision. "I don't know what to do," he says. "I didn't know you were going to ask me to decide anything today; I only wish my wife were here. Can't we wait until she comes back tomorrow?"

Pointing over at Alan thrashing in the bed, the doctor says that she recommends that the procedure be done as soon as possible so that Alan can rest more easily.

"I don't know," says Sollenberger. "I feel like I'm on a roller coaster, me and Alan and the rest of the family on this roller coaster, going up and down and up and down—never on any 'straight ahead' for any given period of time. Alan has been on a roller coaster since the transplant; in the hospital, out of the hospital, on and on, like it will never stop."

The doctor nods politely, signifying some essence of understanding, but studiously avoids the subject obsessing Sollenberger: the quality of life or lack thereof of transplant recipients. Instead, she repeats once again that Alan would be better served with a tracheostomy inserted as soon as possible. "This is not a permanent procedure," she says. "It's completely reversible and it will provide him with much more comfort."

Having not received an answer, the doctor leaves, and Basil Zitelli arrives soon thereafter, outwardly calm and controlled but also recognizably edgy. He obviously believes that the trach will be beneficial to Alan, and is a sensible action, but in his heart he wishes more than anything that this decision, despite its obvious nature, were completely unnecessary. Basil Zitelli wishes that Alan and his father and all the rest of the robust Sollenberger clan were at home on their farm, where they belong, tending to their Guernseys, having only to worry about where to sell their next quart of milk and pound of butter. His face is a mask of embarrassed and compassionate discomfort as he reintroduces the subject of the tracheostomy to Sollenberger.

"I wish I knew what to do," Sollenberger replies. "I wish I knew whether Alan really wants to go through with this stuff anymore, but I don't know."

"I'm not sure that even Alan can answer that question," says Zitelli. "All we know is that he's getting better; that he's fighting a good fight and that he has weathered a great storm. Perhaps his more positive condition is a sign that he has the will and the desire to continue."

"If I had known for one moment," says Sollenberger, "that he was going to be going backward, slipping so far down two or three weeks ago . . ." He pauses, not knowing exactly what he means to say. "It's the frustration. . . ."

"I've never experienced it firsthand," says Zitelli, "but I believe I know what you mean. I can't tell you what's going to happen. No one can tell you."

There is a long silence, as Zitelli stares at Alan in the bed, with his beloved black rubber snake cradled in his arms, while Sollenberger continues to rock in his chair. A nurse comes over and cleans Alan's face of the blood, now dried and crusted, caused by the tube from the ventilator. Alan is not moving, but you know he's not asleep, because his eyelids flicker open from time to time and he eyeballs his father carefully.

"That little girl," Sollenberger suddenly says, pointing at an empty bed two beds down from Alan's. "That little girl who passed on a couple of days ago after five liver transplants? The one in that bed? I think they were all lucky, I mean the family. Maybe they were really lucky. I don't care what you say. At least the agony of not knowing is all over for those people. They finally know what is going to happen to them next and that nothing is going to happen anymore to their little daughter."

"Do you want me to call your wife and ask her?" says Zitelli.

Sollenberger shakes his head. There are tears streaming down his cheeks. He wipes away the tears with the back of his large hand. "I don't know whether I want to mess up her day."

Zitelli nods, continuing to stare at Alan, avoiding the eyes of the crying father, as do I.

"At least he got his toolbox for Christmas," Sollenberger says.

"Alan? Did you get a toolbox?" Zitelli says loudly, with overzealous enthusiasm. "Are you going to help your dad fix his tractor?"

"No," says Sollenberger. "I'm afraid he's going to chop it in half."

"The tracheostomy," said Zitelli, "is made of soft elastic. It won't hurt him. After he gets better and his lungs are clear of fluid, we'll be able to pull it out. The hole that we make in his throat will be healed in twenty-four to forty-eight hours."

"I wish," says Sollenberger as he rocks back and forth in the chair, "that that boy was older, and he could tell me his thoughts."

"We're making progress with Alan," says Zitelli. "We're moving in the right direction."

After a while, Zitelli tells Sollenberger that he will return later to answer any questions. Sollenberger nods, thanking Zitelli for his patience, while continuing his rhythmic rocking.

Later, he says, "I look around and see everybody walking outside in the street or at home. I look around at these people, and I wonder if they know how lucky they are to be healthy and to be alive. I wonder if they've ever walked into this hospital or any place like it and seen what I have seen over the past few years.

"This is the funniest process," says Sollenberger. "This is something that I never imagined could happen. Organ transplantation can kill the family, while the patient," he points at Alan, thrashing and confused in his bed, "goes on and on. And for what? That's what I want to know. Why is this happening to Alan and when is it all going to end?"

Chapter 18

ALTHOUGH he is the second-to-youngest of the GZMU group, and outwardly the most socially reticent, thirty-six-year-old Andrew Urbach feels especially qualified and skillful in communicating devastating information—such as death—to parents and families.

Urbach's mother died four years ago after a ten-year-long illness which began when he was in high school; thus, at an early age, he was made acutely aware of the other side of the doctor-patient relationship and the subtle but vital needs of the family during these painfully crucial periods. The use of the word "skillful" in this context may be disturbing, but doctors do not rely only upon their own sympathetic spontaneity when imparting bad news. Discussing death is as much a part of the profession as is discussing medication, treatment, therapy, and overall good health, Urbach told a group of second-year residents to whom he was lecturing one afternoon. He urged them to develop "a sense of their own style in treating this very difficult event."

Urbach stressed the need to be honest with and direct to parents and families, "and let them know exactly what you are thinking; no tiptoeing around the situation—even if death is only a remote possibility. You might say, 'Have you ever thought what might happen when there are no more medicines to treat your child?' This, at least, might be the beginning of an ongoing dialogue. Or you could say, 'You know, there are a lot of children who suffer through this illness and do very well, but a few do die, and you ought to be aware of it.' "

The actual words are less important than facial expression, tone of voice, and the overall mood created at the moment the family is approached. "I once said to a family, 'I've dealt with a lot of families who have confronted the death of their child in a variety of ways, but I particularly respect the manner in which you have all supported one another.' I said that to a family right after their child had just died, and although the words might not have been the best or the most appropriate, I conveyed a mood and a message to them.

"Sometimes," said Urbach, "I will stand at the child's bedside and say nothing. Sometimes the faith and bond developed between patient and doctor is so strong that my very presence is enough. You have no real ability to predict how families will react under such circumstances, so you just follow your instincts. Families that you expect to be violent will sometimes just sit there and stare straight ahead, while the shock will be too much for those you had expected to be under control."

During that difficult moment when the pediatrician must face the family of a dying child, time seems to go too slow. You begin to notice little bits of paper on the ground, the way the blanket happens to be arranged or wrinkled as it covers the child, the way the nurse stands. Sensory images are enhanced. The mood of the room and the people in it seem larger than life, Urbach said.

I don't know whether the young residents in the room to whom Urbach was speaking could understand, as they slouched straight-faced around a rectangular conference table, nibbling at their lunches, but I understood exactly the eerie and unforgettable scene that Urbach was attempting to portray. In my two years at Children's Hospital, I was only faced with the actuality of death on a few occasions. The first involved a little boy who had shot himself in the head and was rushed in the middle of the night to the Children's ER. The frantic and fruitless efforts of the trauma physicians as they struggled to restore breathing are a slow-motion movie that even today periodically filters through my mind, and the wail of the heartsick mother and grandmother will forever echo in my ears. Just as Urbach explained to the residents, small and unimportant events—sometimes even the silliest of details—become magnified during the tension and drama of the moment. During that night, I remember, the doorknob to the Trauma Room fell off; even now I can hear it crashing to the ground.

Karen Christman, the social worker assigned to the ICU, knows from experience to expect and to respond to thoughts and details that do not seem to be particularly important at the moment. "It's what I've learned from the nurses. Does the family need to sit down? Does the family need to hold the baby? Have all the family members gone into the room to see the child? Do you know where the Kleenex can be found? Sometimes the best thing you can do is to know where the Kleenex are. And things to drink—people will need to drink something in the midst of such devastation."

Christman once heard a SIDS (Sudden Infant Death Syndrome) mother discuss the day her baby died. She and her husband had followed the ambulance to the hospital and endured the shock of suddenly losing their child. "They left the hospital, hours later, and spent an hour in the parking lot looking for their car, because, of course, when they parked it, and climbed out of it, the last thing in their minds was to remember where they were parking. So the final and most vivid memory of the worst day of their lives was wandering in an ugly underground parking lot, trying to figure out how to get home."

Urbach remains a strong believer in the clinical benefits of the autopsy, and he feels that in the long run, the autopsy may well make the experience a little bit easier for the family as well. He cited statistics indicating that autopsies reveal misdiagnosis about 20 percent of the time; the proper diagnosis, of course, might have led to a change in therapy and in prolonged survival. In an additional 20 percent of the cases, autopsies have revealed an unknown secondary diagnosis. Discovering such mistakes and miscalculations enhances knowledge, thus directly benefiting patients and families both scientifically and emotionally.

Urbach said that he sometimes attempts to go to the morgue and observe part of the autopsy, but the experience is quite traumatic. He pauses and ponders the thought momentarily: "I guess 'traumatic' is the wrong word. It's an interesting feeling to take a patient from the first time you have met them, track them through the course of their illness, and then see them for the last time lying on an autopsy table. This is a step beyond death: a very clinical, technical approach to what was once a living, talking human being. The pathologists may not feel that way, however."

Urbach does not mean that pathologists are less sensitive as human beings, only that they will almost never have contact with the patient when he or she is alive. In fact, they are very clinical and enthusiastic about their somewhat shadowed profession.

According to pathology assistants Diane Schneider, who was a biology major in college, and William Devine, a former high school biology teacher, pediatric pathology is more interesting and challenging than adult pathology because there are so many different types and variations of anomalies in children. As an illustration to prove their point, Schneider and Devine will take you for a tour through their heart museum—two thousand hearts soaking in formaldehyde in glass jars, representing syndromes and variations collected by pathologists at Children's since 1953.

Through the years, the Pathology Department has conducted autopsies on about 60 percent of the patients who have died in the hospital, but because of physicians' attitudes toward autopsy the frequency of requests and approvals has gradually declined. Fifteen years ago, the Pathology Department would do as many as two hundred autopsies a year. This year, they expect to conduct only ninety to one hundred procedures.

The Pathology Department is located in a dark corner of the second floor of the old building, totally isolated from the mainstream of the institution. Since the initiation of the liver transplant program, however, a number of parents—people who would have normally never even considered entering this haunting inner sanctum of the hospital—have been coming to visit.

"They want to see their kids' old livers," says Schneider. Comparing the diseased liver, which is often green, shrunken, knobby, and hard, with a normal liver is often therapeutic to parents who may, after the fact, be having second thoughts about the pain and agony their children were forced to endure—despite the success of the transplant. There are three thousand livers in storage in the Pathology Department, catalogued and cross-listed by name, disease, and anomaly in a computer.

"The children will occasionally show up, too," says Devine.

"Last week a little girl from South America who was transplanted last year came down with her folks," says Schneider.

"We gave her gloves, so that she could touch it," said Devine. "She was touching her old liver, the one that used to be in her body, and laughing and screaming, 'Oh my God, my God. This is a trip!' "

At the end of the discussion with the residents, Urbach asks, "When your patient dies, do you go to the funeral, or do you not?"

"It would depend on the relationship with the family," says one resident.

"But if they ask you to go," Urbach says, "then do you go?"

The residents don't know how to answer this question.

"My view," says Urbach, "is that I almost never go. I think that it crosses boundaries that I prefer not to cross. I thank them for the invitation and I say that my thoughts will be with them, but I cannot be there in person. But it's always important to phone them the next day and then send them a handwritten note."

Part IV

Crusade for the Child

O N the wall in the corridor of the Emergency Room, facing the entrances to the nurses' station and the Physicians' Room, there is a chalkboard. Each examination area in the ER is designated with a block in which is printed the last name of the patient and the initials of the physician assuming responsibility. When resident Laurie Penix initials the last empty block, the chalkboard is filled. It is 10 P.M. The evening dashes on ahead of itself in a whizzing and blinding blur.

Penix helps to stabilize a two-year-old rushed to Children's with a "blue spell"—breathing problems. The child, who lived at Children's with a congenital heart defect from the time she was eight hours old through her first five months, is admitted for observation, a fairly unusual occurrence in the ER. ("We've spent more time at Children's Hospital," says the mother, "than in our own home.")

Penix examines a fourteen-year-old transfer from a nearby hospital with "possible appy [appendicitis]." The girl has her name— Peggy—printed in marker on the sole of each shoe. Each time Penix presses on her side, the girl cringes. "I'm sorry, I'm sorry, please understand, I'm sorry," Penix repeats in an annoyed and embarrassed way.

Penix sees a twelve-year-old boy who has accidentally ingested a dose of the tranquilizer Librium. She sees a fifteen-year-old girl with abdominal pains, caused, says Penix, by her menstrual period.

"No," she replies to the girl's question, "Alka Seltzer is for indigestion. Take Tylenol."

Penix performs a spinal tap on a boy suspected of having meningitis. She treats three wheezers in the six-bed OBS (observation) area, one off and on for more than six hours, until he is properly hydrated (the fluid balance is restored). She listens, without laughing, to concerned parents explaining that their pharmacist had recommended phenobarbital to reduce fever in children—an "old wives" treatment.

Meanwhile, Molly O'Gorman examines a child whose mother suspects she swallowed a bobby pin—and arranges for an immediate X-ray. Head nurse Maureen Cusack tells me that working at Children's she's seen all sorts of objects inserted "into every imaginable opening" in a child's body. "I once looked into a kid's ear—and saw these two little eyes bugging out at me. It was a Cootie toy."

Ingestion of poisons is also a large problem at pediatric institutions. Children's Hospital, home of the Pittsburgh Poison Center, is the coordinating body of the National Poison Center Network, which links fifty-four poison information centers and more than two hundred treatment hospitals across the United States. When doctors and nurses in emergency rooms are confronted with a child who has ingested a harmful substance, the Poison Center can be accessed twenty-four hours a day, seven days a week, through a facsimile system that will relay current information about the product, the danger, and the most effective antidotes. Counting inquiries from parents, the Center responds to more than 150,000 calls annually.

Laurie Penix sees a patient with scabies, a highly communicable skin disease caused by a parasite called an itch mite that triggers intense itching. (Later, through the microscope, Bruce Rosenthal shows the residents how the scabies itch mites have burrowed under the child's skin and laid eggs.) Penix sees a patient with Stevens-Johnson syndrome, an even more serious skin eruption. "This kid's face is a disaster area."

O'Gorman greets a four-year-old boy named Jewel, yet another wheezer, for the third time that evening. "I remember you. We're getting to be good friends." Jewel is frightened. Anytime O'Gorman or any of the nurses approaches, he will say, "I'm not going to cry. I promise I won't cry. I promise I'll be good." And then he cries. As the doctors and nurses attempt to get closer, Jewel cries some more.

O'Gorman requests and receives permission from Bruce Rosenthal to use TAC, tetracone adrenalin cocaine, a newly developed local anesthetic for a little girl who requires a dozen stitches for a cut above her eye. "It works great, but there's some concern about a child breathing that stuff in."

Although the transition is subtle, it is quite apparent that the staff has slowly and simultaneously geared up, walking faster, avoiding eye contact with patients and with one another, conversing sparingly, smiling minimally. The casual atmosphere has gradually intensified to a rapid though not full-speed pace. In the back of their mind, they all know that a significant store of energy must always be preserved; Level I trauma (severe auto accidents, drownings, gunshots, etc.) is a constantly looming threat.

Down the hall, in the Ophthalmology Room, John Reed, a visiting resident on pediatric rotation from Presbyterian-University Hospital, is examining a little girl, seventeen months old, with bloody gray discharge leaking from one eye. The mother, perhaps sixteen, says that a neighbor boy stuck a pencil in her daughter's eye.

"When did it happen?"

"Early yesterday."

Reed looks up sharply. "Why did you wait so long?" His voice has a decided edge of annoyance, but the woman doesn't seem to notice, and she answers passively.

"I guess I thought the swelling was going to go down."

Reed attempts to continue the examination, but the child is frightened and in terrible pain, squirming and screaming. After a while, Reed asks the nurse, Marianne Bove, who has rotated from Triage, where she worked earlier that evening, to get a papoose board—sort of a stretcher with Velcro and canvas straps as restrainers.

"Dana, this is a special board with seat belts," says Bove. "We're going to wrap you in a blanket and make you nice and warm."

Reed cleans up the discharge with a Q-Tip. Blood bubbles from behind the eye. Periodically, Reed asks Bove to dim the bright lights so that he can look into the eye with a tiny flashlight. Because of the delicacy of the wound, the examination seems to continue interminably, while the atmosphere in the warm and windowless room grows tense. As Dana screams and squirms, the mother, holding a month-old newborn in her lap, swivels nervously back and forth, rocking in a chair, staring at the wall. Even in the shadowed darkness, the mother rocks, swivels, and stares away from her child, as if in a trance.

"Would you be more comfortable stepping out?" Bove finally asks her.

"Yeah, I would," she says, jumping up.

"We'll come and get you when it's over."

Eventually, Reed decides to summon the ophthalmologist on call at Eye and Ear Hospital, which, along with Presbyterian-University Hospital, is part of the University of Pittsburgh Medical Health Care Division. He also decides to relax the child so that she will be calmer during the examination. A Burger King cup in which a mild sedative has been dissolved is brought in and Dana thirstily drinks it down.

"Thirsty no more," says Bove, caressing the child's ankles.

Dana's eyes are closed when the mother returns to the room fifteen minutes later. She peers down at her daughter. "I guess she's dozing."

Standing at a counter in the corridor, writing on his patient's chart, Reed takes a deep breath: "I was a little short with her, and I shouldn't automatically assume that a parent is at fault in these situations. But that mother knew that the child had been stuck in the eye with the sharp part of a pencil, and to most people that should represent a serious injury. I know I was wrong letting my anger flash like that. It doesn't do any good."

"Anger," says Rosenthal, "is a funny emotion. I mean, not only do I get angry at parents, but also at the kids I am trying to help. The first time I felt this was as a resident during my oncology rotation when I was up every third night with a sick child. When a child finally died, I would experience this great sense of relief—not only for the child but also for myself, because I wouldn't have to crawl out of bed and care for that poor kid anymore.

"Maybe that's why I like emergency medicine so much. I like the fact that I don't have ongoing patient responsibility. You fix people in the ER and send them home. Then there's also the high drama and the gamut of emotions it causes. You can save a life here. You can put in an airway, give blood, resuscitate a child—snatch him out of the jaws of death.

"Being in emergency medicine, there is an exhilaration that for me is on a number of different levels. There is the exhilaration of landing in a helicopter in a parking lot of some community hospital and jumping out while the blades are still spinning, and I feel like Trapper John or something. That's a very egotistical sort of thing, where I sort of envision myself as involved in drama of the highest sense—the TV kind of thing.

"But real exhilaration comes from knowing that you are doing lifesaving, something really tremendous. When you're cutting open a leg to try and find a vein to stick a needle in, trying to intubate someone so you can breathe for them, or pumping on the chest trying to start the heart—that's exhilarating. And if you're successful, it's wonderful. Even if you're not successful, it still can be exhilarating to think that you've tried hard and done your best."

Bruce Rosenthal stresses the importance of preparing the family for the worst when the situation does not look promising. Most people will more readily deal with death in gradual stages of acceptance. "If I can, I will go, or I will send someone out to say, 'We want you to know that things aren't looking good; we're doing all we can. But the situation is tenuous.'

"First I hang crape," says Rosenthal, "and then, if I must, I deliver the message."

"Do you do that often?"

"About a half dozen times a year."

On her way back to the Physicians' Room, after stitching the little girl, Molly O'Gorman crashes head-on into a paramedic rolling a twelve-year-old girl into one of the critical-care rooms. The girl has had her finger accidentally shot off by her brother, who was cleaning his gun. "This is crazy," she tells the paramedic. "I guess it's the weather."

"No," the paramedic replies, "it's the full moon. The loonies are out in full force tonight."

Here are two more paramedics, accompanying a ten-year-old boy with welts on his arms and face. "He stayed out too late, so when he came home, his mother went after him, beat him. Kid ran to a neighbor, who hid him in a closet and wouldn't tell the mother where he was. They contacted the grandfather, but the grandfather lives on the other side of the city, and he didn't sound right over the telephone. I think he was drunk."

"So then?" said Rosenthal.

"They called the police, and that's how we got involved. We wanted to take him in, I mean to here, right away, for an examination, but we all had cold feet because we couldn't get parental consent. The cops were as worried as we were, so they had to call their supervisor for permission. They took pictures and everything before they let us go."

For about ten minutes, the boy is inexplicably left alone, not so much because of the demanding pace of the ER, but more, it seems to me, as I stand in the corridor, because everyone is reluctant and embarrassed to talk with him. Usually, I try to distance myself not only from the patients but also from the doctors and nurses, yet I feel drawn to this youngster—I hurt for him. I walk into his room.

"How you doing?" I say.

The boy is tall and skinny. His clothes are ripped. His feet are dirty, and he sits awkwardly on the examination table, directly under the bright lights of the room and picks his toes.

"I don't know. Okay, I guess."

"I hear you had a rough night."

Now he kind of rolls his eyes and tilts his head, as if he is thinking back and assessing the damage. Then he shrugs, but he does not smile. "I think I'm in trouble."

"Don't worry. There are people here to take care of you."

"Who is that?"

"Nurses, doctors . . ."

"What will they do?"

"You'll be all right," says nurse Kathleen Schenkel, as she walks into the room behind me. "I'm paging the social worker."

The boy nods, but I am not certain he knows exactly what the social worker is or does—or cares. Over the past few months, I have seen infants and toddlers admitted through the ER with cigarette burns behind their ears, radiator burns on their thighs, cuts, bruises, broken bones—all inflicted by parents or guardians. The entire country was stunned by little Lisa Steinberg's shameful death in New York's Greenwich Village, but personnel in emergency rooms in any major urban area in the country are similarly stunned on the average of twice each week. Children also frequently appear in the ER who have been repeatedly sexually molested, and in both cases they seem to cope with the humiliation of the examination and the memories of the frightening events that precipitated it by making themselves not care, by adopting a frightening façade of stark indifference.

As I say goodbye, I can see the boy removing himself from this unfamiliar and threatening atmosphere, putting on his suit of emotionally protective armor. You can poke him, prod him, ask him questions, tell him to inhale, exhale, to open wide and say "ahhhh," and he will follow your instructions to the letter with a glazed-over look of acceptance.

Chapter 20

ASK a prominent philosopher, state leader, cult figure, sports personality—anyone—to pinpoint our nation's most valuable natural resource, and they will invariably name the youth of America. And yet a little more than a century ago children in western countries were treated with thoughtless disregard. Physicians back then were not too knowledgeable, but at least they had some experience and a certain amount of willingness to provide health care to adults. Down through the ages, however, infants and sick children, routinely plagued by wriggling masses of roundworms, among other undiagnosed and neglected maladies, were cared for only by their mothers and/or midwives, who ascribed the most serious of diseases to teething, including fevers, which, when persisting, indicated that children were bewitched.

The American Society for the Prevention of Cruelty to Animals was established in 1866, ten years prior to the establishment of the Society for the Prevention of Cruelty to Children, and the first organized effort to protect a child from abuse (1874) was launched by an ASPCA official, who justified his actions by insisting that a child was also an animal.

Elizabeth Elmer, a Children's Hospital social worker in the middle 1950s who had developed an interest in "failure to thrive" children—those who don't grow or gain weight as a reaction to being neglected—ran into a pediatrician who had just completed a lecture focusing on law and medicine. As an example, he had cited a particularly puzzling case on the infant floor, a little boy, fifteen months old, brought to the hospital by young parents who hadn't remained to be interviewed. "The kid was in a coma," said Elmer, "had bulging fontanels [soft spots], lots of peculiar injuries. The pediatrician said to me, 'Why don't you take a look at this kid, see what you think.'

"I didn't have a lot to do that day, so I went up and asked the nurse about the child and described all the things that the pediatrician had said. She began pulling out these cards from her file, and they all were similar to the child. There were cards for six cases—on one floor, on one random day—before she got done. Most of these parents were never referred to a psychologist, a social worker, or a psychiatrist. The kids were treated and went home. There was no reporting law at that time—not until 1969 in Pittsburgh or in any part of the country."

Pediatrician Mary Carrasco's interest in child abuse was heightened in a similarly spontaneous manner. In the Children's ER as a pediatric resident, and subsequently in a high-poverty clinic on the outskirts of the city where she worked a half dozen years, she began to see an increasing number of abused children and to recognize certain signs and symptoms that hadn't been particularly apparent to her before—a pattern. A parent who is bringing a child into the ER or clinic repeatedly for colds, rashes, and other comparatively insignificant problems might actually be there for another reason.

"Often the issue was not the cold at all. They wanted something else: support—emotional support—from, unfortunately, the pediatrician. And that's often difficult because of time restrictions, as well as expensive." It's ironic to note that many parents on Welfare bring their children to the ER for normal checkups and typical health problems because they cannot afford the $20 charged by a private pediatrician. Yet, because of the cost of the facilities and the personnel on duty, Children's must charge the state a bare minimum of $60 per visit to recoup expenses.

And the system makes serious counseling nearly impossible. "When I was in the ER or at the clinic, I did what I was told to do, which was, when someone came in and said, 'Well, I'm going so crazy I may well kill my child tomorrow,' I'd say, 'I have twenty patients in the waiting room and I don't have an hour to spend with you. Would you be able to come back tomorrow afternoon?' And they'd say, 'Yes.'

"But they wouldn't come back, because to identify the behavior issue as something they had to come back and talk about was too threatening. It was much easier to bring the child in and say, 'This child has a cold,' when you could see that the child's cold was not the issue at all. They would come in for support."

One of the principal and telltale signs of serious abuse are multiple bone injuries. "These occur in succession, not all at once," says Elmer. "It isn't like an automobile accident, which may happen simultaneously to many parts of your body. It's as though today you were hit on your arm and got a little fracture, tomorrow your leg is wrenched, or a month from now something else happens. On an X-ray, you can see these lesions, in different healing stages, and that's how we identify them."

This process of recognizing variations in the time of healing was developed in 1946 by a pediatric radiologist at Babies Hospital in New York, John Caffey, who subsequently joined Children's Hospital of Pittsburgh after his mandatory retirement at age sixty-five. Caffey was extremely encouraging and helpful to Elmer, who was to conduct a landmark "50 Family Study," one of the very first examinations of the victims of child abuse, which demonstrated that child abuse was, even in the 1950s, at near-epidemic proportions.

Recently, Elmer and a colleague conducted a followup study of twenty of the original fifty children she was able to locate (eight had died in childhood, presumably from the effects of abuse), most of whom were so young during the study that they did not realize that they were abused. "There was one woman, however, who was abused consistently up until the time she was about four. She had kept all the newspaper clippings and brought them all out, and kind of wallowed in being abused.

"Out of the group of twenty, twelve were unmarried and nine had no children. And two of them said, 'Well, I'd like to have children, but I just thought I shouldn't take the chance.' So even if they didn't know about themselves literally, they had recognized that maybe they had some impulse or predilection to not treat kids well."

Elmer eventually founded the Parental Stress Center, where abused babies who had been placed in foster homes could be reunited for a trial training period with their natural parents. The Center has expanded its activities and moved to quarters outside of Children's Hospital but maintains a close affiliation.

Carrasco also founded a drop-in center for parents who feel sudden anxiety and/or the need to speak to a counselor or to be in a protective and nonthreatening atmosphere. "We have child-care workers and foster grandparents who greet parents at the door as if they've come into a home." Drop-in centers are becoming increasingly evident in low-income neighborhoods across the United States, but one of Carrasco's objectives at her newly established Family Intervention Center (FIC) at Children's Hospital is to establish a similar center in middle- and upper-middle-class areas. Studies show that there are few class distinctions in child abuse. What distinguishes cases of abuse in varying social and cultural strata is the income for attorneys and private counselors who can often mask the crime.

Born and educated in Bombay, India, Carrasco had been troubled by child abuse at a very young age. She explains that her countrymen of the lower classes, such as construction workers, would often take their children on the job with them, to help or because they had no other way to occupy them. "If the children did something wrong or got in the way, it was not uncommon for the parents to beat them right out on the street. I would get very upset when I saw an adult hurting a child, but my mother and father wouldn't let me involve myself. They would tell me that it wasn't the parents' fault for hurting that child. They would tell me that you had to change the conditions that made the abuse a possibility.

"The funny thing is," says Carrasco, "if you talk to people in India—physicians, pediatricians, whatever—they will tell you that child abuse is an American phenomenon. It's all around them, more visible than anything occurring in the United States, and yet they are blind to it."

It would be unfair to say that Indians, or those of any other nationality or culture, are singularly blind to child abuse, for it has been a heretofore unrecognized international disgrace. In 1987 in the state of Pennsylvania, there were 21,000 reports of suspected child abuse, with 7,000 actually substantiated. Half of the incidents were sexual injuries inflicted by parents. Forty-four abused children died, but experts say that there are many more tragedies that for one reason or another are never reported.

"It's an intriguing thing in our society that we haven't really recognized the needs of kids. We've been concentrating for the last twenty-five years on the elderly," says Robert Sweeney of the National Association of Children's Hospitals and Related Institutions (NACHRI). Sweeney cites the federally funded health-care benefits originally set up principally for orphaned or dependent children— "a single-parent situation, mother not married or abandoned." Today, according to Sweeney, half of the money allocated for this purpose is being diverted to the elderly. In fact, taking into consideration the other programs funded under the same umbrella, approximately 85 percent of all of the Medicare health-care dollars is spent on people over sixty-five.

Ned Zechman, president of Children's Hospital, says that he is not against federally funded programs for the elderly, but he insists that Congress, for too long, has been one-sided. "Today, we have finally made a group of our population—the elderly—free from concern about catastrophic health-care costs. That's wonderful, but what makes an elderly person more vulnerable to catastrophic health care than a child? One could be cynical and say the difference is a child does not vote and the Gray Panthers do. The Association of Retired People (AARP) spearheads a very strong lobby.

"The children we take care of come from young parents who are starting out in their careers. They haven't amassed their fortunes yet, bought their homes; they're in their first jobs. They don't vote regularly. All you have to do is look at a demographic study of who votes and who doesn't to know that the older you get, the more you vote. I'm not against Medicare at all, but I don't know that those people are any more deserving than the people who are at the other end of the age spectrum.

"If you look at it on a cost/benefit ratio basis, it would seem to me that one could make an argument that the investment in a child and in preventive health care, and taking care of that chronic illness that the child was born with, is worth an awful lot more to society in the long run than the tremendous amount of money we spend on somebody's last three or four days of life."

The value of the child to society and to the future of our nation is an issue repeatedly stressed by Marian Wright Edelman, founder of the prestigious and activist Children's Defense Fund. "The Committee for Economic Development recently recognized that children are a shrinking proportion of our population as it ages, and that unless preventative investment in early childhood is made a national policy, our future work force will be disproportionately poor, unhealthy, untrained, and uneducated, and we will not be able to be competitive in the global arena."

Zechman, forty, one of the youngest chief executive officers of a major health-care institution in the United States, is responsible for governmental relations, fund-raising, and legislation affecting pediatrics generally and Children's specifically in Harrisburg, the

Pennsylvania state capital, and in Washington. He says that 40 percent of U.S. children between the ages of one and four were not immunized against measles, mumps, polio, or rubella in 1984, even though "one dollar spent on immunization can save ten dollars in 'down-the-road' medical costs. Thirty-four percent of U.S. pregnant women are getting very little, if any, prenatal care. But we are told that the danger of a low-birth weight baby is six times higher for a mom who did not get prenatal care—and that baby is forty times more likely to suffer complications, to fail, and to die in the first few months of life."

Zechman points out that there are 11 million children—17 percent of the population under eighteen—with neither public nor private health insurance. There are now approximately eleven deaths of children for each thousand born in this country. The United States is an embarrassing nineteenth on the world list of infant mortality rates, while Japan, which was seventeenth in 1955, is on top of the list today. A study conducted by Brown University demonstrated that "by age four, children 'at risk' drop by as much as 30 points on intelligence tests compared with well-nurtured 'low-risk' children."

Throughout the next few years, because of Children's Hospital's centennial anniversary, Zechman will be making public appearances on both a local and national level attempting to improve the condition or the "state of the child." New York Governor Mario Cuomo has tagged the 1990s as the "Decade of the Child," while Zechman has launched the "Crusade for the Child"—a write-in campaign to spotlight and support the National Commission on Children. This Commission was established in December 1987 to study and monitor child health-care issues and to hold public hearings throughout the United States in order to submit a consensus report—with recommendations for vital improvements—sometime in 1990.

Another influential interest group is the American Academy of Pediatrics, founded in 1930 by thirty pediatricians who met in Detroit in response to the need for an independent pediatric forum. Today membership is nearing 36,500. The academy has long been active and effective in publicizing and advocating solutions to health-care problems plaguing America's young people. Its current president, pediatrician Birt Harvey, sixty, of Stanford University, also a fellow at the Kaiser Family Foundation, has dedicated great time and effort toward the formation of a national child health policy, which at this moment does not exist in this country.

"We tend to respond to whatever group can exert the most pressure toward having a specific need met, or we respond based upon crises that arise in this country," says Harvey. As an example, children in America with end-stage renal disease have been adequately covered by federally-funded insurance, but for those kids with a number of other chronic diseases, there is no coverage at all. "There's no cohesion to our thinking, no long-term planning. All the programs are categorical. If a child fits into the right niche, he's going to be covered.

"Also, Medicaid is administered by the states, which may provide differing benefits. So a child in one state who has a certain illness may get very good coverage; in another state, he won't be eligible at all because the benefits are at a different level of family income. In some states, you're allowed to be hospitalized only twelve days, no matter what your disease might be. In other states, you get much more complete coverage. That's crazy; that's not fair to kids. Kids didn't ask to be born to one set of parents or in one part of the country. They deserve equal care."

Harvey says that one of the academy's primary goals "is to establish a White House adviser on children. There's nobody on staff who pays attention to or advocates for children." Another objective is to convince the Department of Health and Human Services to examine "the diversity and multiplicity of children's programs and to see if they couldn't be organized more effectively so they're not so separated within the federal bureaucracy. In [the Department of] Agriculture, there's WIC (Women/Infants/Children), there's the school lunch and breakfast. And similarly in Education, there are early childhood education for the handicapped and a number of additional programs that are primarily health-related.

"There are also different eligibility requirements for each program. And in most cases the woman has to go and spend a half a day laboring over the most complex questionnaires to become eligible. This can be a humiliating experience, too, because very often the eligibility-intake workers, rather than feeling that their job is to assist people, try to keep people out of the system. The people who apply really feel degraded by the process."

In addition to standardizing eligibility requirements, the academy is attempting to make Americans aware of the positive ways in which other nations regard and treat their mothers and children. "In many European countries, if a woman is pregnant, she goes to the head of a line waiting for a bus. In France and in most other European countries, there is maternity leave when needed. If a woman has a high-risk pregnancy, she receives money in support, and health-care workers are provided to assist her. There are governmental subsidies for children in Europe and in Canada—automatically.

"There are only two developed nations in this world," says Harvey, "where there is no financial access to care for all children. The United States is one, and South Africa is the other. I don't know what that tells you, but it says something significant to me."

Chapter 21

COMING to the Family Inter-
vention Center's (FIC) sexual-abuse clinic from the detention facility
in which she temporarily lived, Sylvia, a twelve-year-old girl, was
well-scrubbed and neat, except for her hair, which sprouted out in
jagged points in all different directions. Sylvia's mother, who has
been institutionalized for most of her life, gave over her daughter's
custody to an aunt, says the counselor, "and it was the aunt's para-
mour who was the perpetrator."

"And when the mother is not institutionalized, what happens to
her?"

"She stays with the aunt also, locked upstairs in the attic."

The counselor seems to have a good relationship with Sylvia,
although he continually warned us, as he leafed through the file,
that she was a very dangerous person. He limped when he walked,
and later, while Mary Carrasco was examining Sylvia in private, he
told me that the reason he was limping was that Sylvia had been
fighting him through most of the week and that yesterday he had
had to dedicate most of the afternoon to holding her down. Later I
told this to Carrasco, who replied that sometimes she questions the
counselors themselves, suspecting that people go into these very
low-paying jobs in order to satisfy their own urges for a more violent
lifestyle.

The counselor talked bitterly about the system and how difficult
it is to get anything done. He said that his was a thirty-day center

(a center designed for short stays; no more than a month), and he had been trying to get this girl into Mayview, which is a psychiatric hospital, where she could get the help that she needed, but she had been with them for four months, because the system moves so slowly.

He blamed the disintegration of Pittsburgh's steel industry for many of the problems that he and his colleagues had to deal with. Young people could not get jobs and they ended up with drugs and alcohol and nothing else to do but watch television and make babies. He predicted the worst for Sylvia. In one way or another, in some half-hearted fashion, she'll be cared for by the system until she's eighteen, and then she'll be set free to make babies—just like her mother. And these babies will be abused, just as Sylvia was, and just as her mother was. "It's a never-ending cycle," the counselor says. "It gets me sick."

Throughout the examination, Sylvia refuses to provide any information regarding her sexual activities and, as a matter of fact, has a difficult time remembering why she was referred here and when the events precipitating her visit occurred. Her attention remained exclusively focused on her height and weight, to which she responded incredulously, as if she could not believe that she was five feet, five inches tall and nearly 127 pounds. "Wow! Can you believe it! That's impossible!"

Following Sylvia were two little girls, Patricia and Anna, three and five years old, respectively, from a small town thirty miles southwest of Pittsburgh, who had been sexually abused by their father. Just as Carrasco had predicted ("These people desperately need an authority figure to talk with"), the mother, upon the very first question, exploded in an animated fashion, talking about her husband, the environment in which he was born and raised, and how awful and terrible the husband's sister had turned out, having sometimes seven lovers simultaneously. She talked about how cruel her husband had been to her—not abusive but cruel. How he had denied sex to her on occasion, and teased her with sex, promising and then withdrawing.

At the end of the interview, the mother retreated to the waiting area, but then in perhaps three minutes she returned and asked to see Carrasco once again. Back in the room, facing Carrasco across a tiny table, she launched into a story about returning one day from work and discovering little Anna crying softly and running in circles around the living room. She was clutching something tightly in her hand, and when the mother pried loose her fingers, she found a piece of glass. "She kept running around and running around, showing this glass, and her hand was bleeding. And every time I said, 'What happened? Can I help you? What happened? What happened?,' Anna replied, 'I'm a big girl now. I can take care of myself.'"

The mother went upstairs and found her husband sleeping on the water bed with their younger daughter, side by side. And although nothing much was said at the time about the piece of glass, the mother never forgot the incident, and when she discovered that her husband was abusing her babies, it all came back to her. In the back of her mind, the mother had always feared that her husband had inserted that piece of glass in his daughter's vagina.

"I guess I need assurance that this really hasn't happened," the mother concludes.

"Don't worry," says Carrasco. "There was definitely some sort of penetration, but I see no evidence of any permanent damage, nothing that could have been caused by a piece of glass."

Later, I read part of the social worker's interview with Anna. Here are some quotations from that report:

"I asked her why she thought that her father did that to her, and she stated, 'Maybe he didn't know what he was doing.'"

"I questioned her about being asleep or awake when the alleged abuse occurred. She indicated, 'Sometimes I would pretend that I was sleeping, but I really wasn't. When bad things happen, you like to think they are happening in a dream.'"

That morning, I asked Carrasco how she managed, week after week, to hear the raw and intimate details, to subsequently see the faces behind the horror stories and not be seriously affected by them.

"Well," she replied, "it's not that I feel unmoved, but a person in my position has to come to realize that you cannot make an impact on every case."

I asked her if there wasn't a danger in being so blasé that you could lose effectiveness.

"I guess that can happen. But the fact of the matter is that if we got more upset about each case, we would not get as much done. In my experience, when I have allowed myself to get involved, I have achieved less for the family and the child."

This was a rare leisurely morning. A number of the families scheduled were either delayed or had not shown up, so Carrasco was making phone calls in search of experienced therapists to work with FIC on a part-time basis. Between calls, she was explaining the difficulty in locating appropriate personnel. Her advertisements had triggered eighty applications, many from people who, although technically qualified, with impressive published papers and graduate degrees, seemed unacceptable for one reason or another. She recently turned down a candidate who had written her dissertation on the problems of midlife crisis. "Now what does that have to do with assessing child abuse in the emergency room of a pediatric institution?"

Her most promising candidate to date, at least on paper, a forty-year-old male with significant on-the-job experience, had indicated an abnormally strong tendency to protect the alleged perpetrator. During their interview he explained to Carrasco that he went to great lengths to understand and empathize with the point of view of the perpetrator. "He would try to work himself up in a manner that the perpetrator worked himself up, to the point of literal sexual arousal," said Carrasco. "Needless to say, he wasn't for us."

While we're talking, the newly hired full-time child psychologist, Judy Krynski, enters the room to announce that the next appointment had finally arrived, a ten-year-old girl who has been sexually abused by her grandfather. Carrasco quickly departs to conduct the physical part of the examination, then returns within twenty minutes, confirming that the girl was indeed sexually abused. "But it isn't clear whether the grandfather is still living with the family. I know that the father is gone, but I couldn't get the girl to talk about the grandfather. We have to find out if he is still on the premises. The mother says no, but I'm not certain I believe her."

Also, Carrasco has discovered two bruises on the girl's back. "She claims that she keeps falling off her bed, because it's very narrow, landing on an electrical outlet that extends from the wall. But I suspect something else."

Krynski picks up a clipboard and disappears into the examination room. The child, whose name is Andrea, is tall and gangly, with a long blond ponytail. She's wearing pink socks, a pink sweater, high-top tennis shoes with rainbow laces, and black horn-rimmed glasses, and she's chomping on a big wad of gum. As the interview progresses, Andrea chomps down harder and harder on the gum.

Krynski begins by talking about Andrea's birthday, which is evidently coming up.

"What kind of party did you have last year?"

"A pool party with a blow-up pool, but I could only invite one friend to come."

Slowly, Krynski brings the situation around to the subject in question. Krynski has a soft smooth voice, kind of like a female Mr. Rogers.

"Who lives in your family?"

"My mom, my brothers, and me," says Andrea.

"What about your dad?"

"He don't live there."

"When was the last time you've seen him?"

"About a week ago."

"I understand," says Krynski, pausing, "that Grandpop used to live with you. When was the last time you saw him?"

"I don't know."

"I know that this is hard for you to talk about, Andrea, but . . ."

"I'm scared," says Andrea.

"Scared of what might happen?"

"Yeah."

"I have heard that your grandfather touched you in the private genital area."

Andrea nods her head in acknowledgment.

"Did it happen once?"

"Twice," says Andrea.

"Where was it? Where did it happen?"

"In the bedroom."

"What time did it happen?"

"In the dark."

"You were in pajamas?"

"Nightgown."

"What did your grandfather have on when he came up to your bed?"

Andrea is leaning forward now, speaking in a very soft babylike whisper, kind of scrunching up her shoulders and stooping down over the little interviewing table. A plastic necklace, a rainbow of colors similar to her shoe laces, has gotten tangled in her ponytail. She untangles it and wraps it around her hand.

"Did your grandfather say anything to you as he approached the bed?" asks Krynski.

"He told me not to tell anybody."

"It would be helpful if you could tell me exactly what he did," says Krynski.

"He laid down next to me in the bed."

"The covers were pulled down?" asks Krynski.

Andrea nods.

"Did he touch your genital area? Is that what you call it?"

"I call it private parts," says Andrea.

"Well, Andrea, in your private parts, we actually have two parts," says Krynski. "A front part and then a hole in the back part called the vagina. Which part did he touch you?"

"Both parts," says Andrea.

"Did you lie there without moving?"

Andrea nods.

"What did you do?"

"I cried."

"Did you feel that that was the right thing for him to do?"

"No," she answers.

"When he finished, did he leave?" asks Krynski.

"He stayed."

"He stayed?"

"Because he shared the bedroom with me."

"Was that the first time it happened?"

Andrea nods.

"What happened the second time?"

"Same thing," says Andrea.

"Was grandfather drinking?"

"Yes. Rum and coke."

"What does he do when he has a lot to drink?"

"He yells at Mom and calls her dirty names."

"What does your mother do when this happens?"

"She tells me to go to bed."

"You mentioned that Grandfather moved out. Do you know where he's gone?"

"No."

"Right now in your house without Grandfather being there, do you feel safer?"

"Yes."

"Dr. Carrasco mentioned that you have two bruises on your back. How did that happen?"

"Fell off the bed and landed on a plug."

"Dr. Carrasco says that the bruises look suspicious, and she doesn't think that they happened in exactly that way. Do you have anything to tell me?"

"No."

"How do you and your mom get along?"

"Good."

"Are you well behaved at home?"

She doesn't answer.

"How does Mom discipline you?"

"She yells at me."

"Does she ever hit you?"

"No."

"How about your grandpop. Didn't he hit you?"

She nods. "With a wooden paddle," she says.

"On your backside?"

"Yes."

"When would he paddle you?"

"When I didn't listen to my mom."

"Did she want him to do it?"

"No."

"How did he do it?"

"He held my arms down, and he hit me."

"And now that's stopped?" says Krynski.

"Yes, because the paddle broke," says Andrea.

"Were you responsible? Did you break it?" asks Krynski.

"I wish I could have," says Andrea, "but I didn't."

Andrea leaves the room now, and Krynski brings the mother in. The mother is a tall, tough-looking woman with a blue plaid flannel shirt, and short, stringy brown hair. She has a very masculine-looking face with a pained expression. In a very deep voice, she says that she suffers from terrible tension headaches; she has one at this moment, in fact.

"How are things going at home?" asks Krynski.

"She's still a brat," says the mother. "Ever since Dad left, she back-talks everybody, and she only gets better when her dad comes back."

"How long has her dad been gone?" says Krynski.

"About a month."

"She mentioned that sometimes Grandfather would hit her with a paddle."

"Sometimes," the mother admits, "but not often. The only time I personally use a belt is when she gets out of hand."

"Andrea said that your dad used to drink a lot and that you two always fought."

"Oh, me and him," says the mother, "we used to have our fights when he drinks. I just ignore him when he starts to yell and scream, and sooner or later he falls asleep on the floor beside my bed."

"It sounds like you are under a lot of stress," says Krynski.

"I am, definitely," says the woman.

"Was your separation from your husband a mutual decision?"

"Not a mutual decision," says the mother. "He just come home, packed his clothes, and left. Two years ago he left me also. I was drinking very heavily back then because my sister had just died. But I'm not drinking heavily anymore."

"But you are drinking somewhat?" asks Krynski.

"Oh, once a week—if that," the mother replies.

"Andrea mentioned that she fell from the bed and hit a plug—an outlet."

"Yeah, I watched her do it. She was running away from me, because I went after her, because she was mouthing off at me."

"What is your source of income?"

"DPA [Department of Public Assistance]."

"Have your headaches increased recently?"

"Significantly."

Later, back in the consultation room, Krynski and Carrasco agree that they will have to continue to watch this family situation closely. They are not certain whether the grandfather has, in fact, left the house, but they believe that the bruises on the child's back were caused by the events the mother described. Carrasco says, "The fact that the mother finally blamed herself to a certain extent is significant to me. She wasn't trying to hide anything after she got to talking. She remained up-front."

Chapter 22

ALTHOUGH physicians, psychologists, social workers, and health-care administrators are often powerless to protect the child against society and the complicated and unwieldy system designed to protect them, they do realize that in many respects children are equally vulnerable within the sheltered confines of the hospital or medical center.

According to the American Hospital Association, more than 60 percent of its member hospitals have ethics or human rights committees to review treatment decisions by the staff, or a philosopher or ethicist in residence available to all hospital or university personnel and to patients and families for consultations and/or to act as liaison and, if necessary, arbitrator between conflicting groups.

Children's Hospital's Human Rights Committee (HRC), once called the Institutional Review Board, also reviews all research protocols for any research that is proposed involving subjects in the hospital. No research whatsoever—no matter how harmless it may seem—is permitted without the approval of the Human Rights Committee, which meets from 2:00 P.M. to 6:00 P.M. on the third Thursday of every month. From May 1, 1987, through April 30, 1988, the committee, composed of medical and administrative personnel along with one private practice pediatrician and one clergyman unaffiliated with Children's, reviewed 144 renewal applications for research in progress. Of the 122 new proposals also reviewed during that period, 43 were approved outright, after discussion, and only four were disapproved. The remaining 64 were also eventually approved, but with "contingencies."

Some of the research protocols submitted to the HRC are simple and straightforward, such as one recent case that analyzed "the effectiveness of written instructions" in relation to parental treatment and compliance of the patient. Others are more complicated, including a proposal entitled "The Role of Alcohol in Adult/Child Interactions," in which the alcoholic drink of choice is given in increasingly large measures to adult volunteer subjects during a prescribed period while the behavior of a child-actor, employed for the experiment, becomes more difficult to control. The scene is videotaped and observed from the next room via a see-through mirror.

Although sounding quite bizarre, the object of the study is to shed light on the interactions between parents with substance abuse problems and their children, providing insight into a number of areas, including events that precipitate child abuse and/or cause behaviors that can lead to developmental delay (such as depression, withdrawal, etc.) in the child. There was a long discussion, in which a gamut of possible problems were analyzed, from the possibility of harm inflicted upon the child-actor by a potentially alcoholically enraged adult, to the liability of the hospital in the event that the adult injured himself during his or her "drunkenness" or on the way home afterward. One of the investigators gave testimony, and the project was finally approved.

Concern for subjects involved in experimentation also includes animals. Both Children's Hospital and the University of Pittsburgh have separate animal laboratory facilities, along with animal rights (Animal Research and Care) committees, charged with the responsibility of overseeing the use of animals in scientific experimentation: pigs, cows, lambs, and especially dogs (primarily beagles, because of size and availability) are frequently employed in surgical trials. Before Thomas Starzl attempted a historic multivisceral (multiple-organ) transplant, the surgery and immunosuppression were tested on a number of animals, including one pig that survived nearly three months.

Contrary to popular belief, animals are not nearly as durable as humans, while from an economic and practical point of view, the post-op care of animals cannot be as thorough and diligent. A three-month animal survivor was sufficient evidence to persuade the HRC to allow Starzl to attempt the procedure on a child on a one-time trial basis, especially considering the fact that the patient was in imminent jeopardy. If and when Starzl wanted to attempt a series of multivisceral transplants, however, a new HRC protocol would be required, based on the knowledge and insight provided by the transplant team's experience. The HRC also has the authority to permit physicians to use experimental medication on a one-time "emergency" basis.

Approval by the HRC with "contingencies" for animal or human subjects ranges from the esoteric scientific (questions concerning dosage of a prescribed medication) or an adjustment in surgical procedures to more down-to-earth considerations, such as the exact wording of the informed consent form, which must accompany each research protocol, to be signed by the child's parents. When Jeffrey Malatack submitted his protocol for the bone marrow transplant program he was launching, for example, the HRC requested that Malatack replace the phrase "sucked out" with the word "withdrawn," in the phrase "bone marrow will be sucked out from our child's hip bones." In another paragraph, the HRC asked Malatack to indicate the "approximate level of risk of cardiac or respiratory arrest leading to death" while the child donating the marrow was under anesthesia. Malatack thus defined for the parents the risk of cardiac arrest as one chance in 100,000.

According to the federal regulations concerning research on normal children, established in March 1983, all four of the following conditions must be established for the research to be approved:

- the risk must represent a minor increase over minimal risk;
- the intervention or procedure must present experiences to subjects that are reasonably commensurate with those inherent in their actual or expected medical, dental, psychosocial, or educational situations;
- the intervention or procedure must be likely to yield generalizable knowledge about the subject's disorder or condition, which is of vital importance for the understanding or amelioration of the subject's disorder or condition; and
- adequate provisions must be made for soliciting the assent of the children and permission of their parents or guardians.

Joel Frader, a pediatrician who has a master's degree in sociology, explains that there are four elements to be considered under the umbrella of informed consent, beginning with "disclosure." How much information is actually disclosed to the patient and/or family about the research project? In terms of comprehension, how much does the patient and/or parent understand of what will happen, how the experiment will work? The third aspect is freedom from coercion: Has the patient and/or family been pressured to comply in any conceivable manner? The last consideration has to do with competence: Is the patient or family who has been asked to make the decision truly competent to make that decision? This latter category includes mental illness or intellectual impairment, negative effects from substance abuse, as well as tension and stress from a long and fearful hospital siege.

The term "informed consent" applies primarily to adult patients and to parents of children considered to be minors under the law. But children can have some control over their own fate even if they are minors. While parents can give permission or consent for research, competent children, at the same time, must also give their "assent," meaning that they can object to being subjects in the research protocol. Federal guidelines suggest that a normal child of seven would be qualified to give assent, but because many psychiatrists argue that children mature differently, most doctors and/or human rights committees will make their own determination based on the patient in question.

Frader relates "assent" to a child's understanding of life, death, and morality. He points out that the influential child psychologist Jean Piaget has said that children can understand death by age nine, but if they have been chronically ill for a long period of time, they are capable of understanding death as early as four. "Also," says Frader, "the Catholic church has a belief that by age seven a child is capable of moral distinction."

The words "moral" and "distinction" are paramount in most of the problems Frader confronts in his role of medical ethicist. During the same May through April period, Frader conducted or participated (with two other HRC members) in eight separate human rights consultations, attempting to understand, articulate, and mediate practical, moral, and ethical disagreements between parents and their children's doctors. One of the most complicated of the cases confronted by Frader and his colleagues dealt with a child who was permanently respirator-dependent.

The child, four months old at the time of the HRC consultation, was transferred to Children's Hospital on the first day of life because of an inability to eat or breathe. Since then, the child had required continuous mechanical ventilation and a gastrostomy tube placement. She is only slightly responsive to her environment. "All physicians involved," Frader and two colleagues reported to the HRC, agree that the likelihood of neurologic improvement is "vanishingly" small. "We should not expect her to acquire language or any communicative skills. While she apparently feels pain, there is no evidence that she can or will experience pleasure. To use a somewhat muddy concept, she will not become a person." The dilemma for the hospital, however, rests with the mother, a former nurse, who remains unalterably opposed to the discontinuation of ventilator support.

Although in disagreement with the mother (who would not speak directly with the HRC), the HRC report does attempt to present her point of view: "One could simply say that accepting the mother's strong investment in continuing ventilation, though perhaps ill arrived at, at least in some way preserves the custom of respecting family autonomy. Indeed, one could claim that the mother's emotional stability and/or personal beliefs would be cruelly impinged upon by an imposed termination of treatment and the baby's death." But the consultants concluded that "while we can agree that our approach to the mother should be gentle and humane," the hospital is under no obligation to accept the mother's decision.

Frader and all the other members of HRC, as well as all the other parties involved, will accept the mother's decision, however, no matter what the consequences, because of fear of negative publicity and long and time-consuming legal entanglements. At the same time, the consultants also urged the committee to consider the points of view of other people who are necessarily victims of such a case, including the medical and nursing personnel.

"This can be emotionally draining," says Frader, "a violation of conscience, and a waste of their time and energy. The hospital and its community have an interest in seeing that the resources of the institution are employed reasonably—i.e., not squandered on applications doomed to fail. Moreover, in this particular situation, we see a matter that goes beyond the claims on the general pool of time, money, equipment, et cetera available to care for those in need. Here we face the distinct possibility that another patient, clearly a potential beneficiary of the expertise and facilities available, may be turned away precisely because we are devoting resources to this infant's nonbeneficial treatment."

In December 1987, I sat in on a special meeting of an HRC

subcommittee convened to address this problem. Also present, in addition to members of the committee, were the president of the hospital, Ned Zechman, the medical director, William Donaldson, and Ann Thompson, the director of the hospital's intensive-care facilitie.. After a long and intense debate, examining all the options related to the situation, the subject was tabled. Frader was asked to discuss the problem with colleagues at other institutions and attempt to rally their support, while Thompson and the hospital's legal counsel were to investigate possible legislative (state and federal) options. One year later, the subcommittee had not been reconvened, and neither Frader nor Thompson expected that new and viable solutions to the problem could or would be put forth in the foreseeable future.

"No one is willing to expend the energy it will take to get the job done—it's a full-time effort," Thompson comments. "And no one is willing to make themselves so vulnerable in a public debate between a loving mother and a group of physicians and a hospital bent upon taking her child's life, no matter how legitimate the reasons." The cause may be just, but the cost in time and reputation would be far too great a sacrifice.

Chapter 23

BRUCE ROSENTHAL was still on duty in the Emergency Room a little after midnight when a call came in about a three-year-old boy who had shot himself in the face with his father's .357 magnum. Usually, radio calls regarding trauma from medics en route to Children's are accepted by the hospital dispatcher and relayed to the trauma command surgeon, who captains the trauma team. But this was a direct communication from the ambulance speeding to the hospital to a radio in the ER normally used by EMTs to talk with physicians about critical medical problems. "I was carrying a walkie-talkie," said Rosenthal, "and I immediately radioed Communications that we had a gun wound to the face, ETA five minutes, and I just started telling the nurses, 'Okay, I know you're tired, but let's get moving.' "

Children's Hospital of Pittsburgh is one of Pennsylvania's twenty-one designated trauma centers accredited by the Trauma Systems Foundation of Pennsylvania (the only other designated pediatric trauma center is Children's Hospital of Philadelphia). All significant pediatric injuries within a 100-mile radius are transported directly to the Children's Emergency Room. There, in addition to the regular staff, a trained surgical team, with anesthesiologists, respiratory therapists, and other essential specialties such as orthopedics or neurosurgery, is on call twenty-four hours a day. A Level I trauma is life-threatening, whereas a Level II trauma, although quite serious, is not, at least not at the moment the child is admitted.

For Level III traumas—cuts and bruises—the trauma team is usually not employed.

The cornerstone of trauma is known as "the golden hour"—the first hour after the incident, when, despite injury, the body is usually able to sustain itself. "The golden hour" is a term initially developed by medics who cut their teeth in Korea and Vietnam. It is ideally divided into three equal increments: Twenty minutes for the EMT (Emergency Medical Technician) to arrive on the scene; twenty minutes for assessment and stabilization; twenty minutes for transport to the trauma center. The sooner the injured child can be attended to by the trauma team, the greater the likelihood that child's life will be saved.

"I used to give this lecture comparing trauma today to the great plague of the Middle Ages," says Marc Rowe, chief of Surgical Services at Children's and founder of the Benedum Pediatric Trauma Program, named for the foundation which in 1984 donated the $722,000 three-year start-up grant. "Trauma is the most common cause of death for children and adults up to age thirty—three times as common as cancer or heart disease."

Trauma, says Rowe, is a surgical problem, and an emergency room is a medical facility. "That's why we don't want emergency rooms in the community handling trauma, because if you walk into a community hospital emergency room, what you'll run into is a medical doctor, and medical doctors are good for heart attacks, for fevers, sore throats, those kinds of things. But if you've been in a car accident, you want somebody who knows surgical procedures; you want a surgeon, you want a surgical support team—and you want them fast. In critical situations, your life depends on it." The gunshot boy was one of 600 traumas confronted in 1988 by the Children's Hospital trauma team. Of the 100,000 accidental deaths in the U.S. each year, 25,000 of them are pediatric.

Within five minutes the entire Level I trauma team—emergency room doctors, trauma team surgeons, nurses, and respiratory therapists—have all gathered in Trauma Room 1. The temperature in the room has been increased by ten degrees in case the child is suffering from hypothermia; drug cabinets are unlocked, swung open. Nurses hurriedly gown one another, then gown and glove the surgeons as they walk through the Trauma Room door. White latex gloves snap into place. The anesthesiologist prepares his medications and intubation equipment. A nurse sits at a corner desk, ready to receive the vital signs dictated by the command surgeon, who is last to arrive. David Lloyd, recruited to Children's by Marc Rowe from his rural hospital in South Africa—a hospital founded by his father—seems to be completely calm.

"One thing I learned from my father has to do with his Zulu nickname—Mpefene, which means 'one who hurries slowly.'

"So I never panic," says Lloyd. "My father always told me, when things are going bad, take a deep breath, and count to ten. Put all emotional thoughts behind you."

He motions behind him to the members of his team. Senior surgical fellow Steve Teich is clapping his gloved hands together, snapping his fingers, but most everyone else, eight nurses and doctors circling the operating table, are waiting quietly, arms folded, staring at each other idly. As the seconds tick by, the tension in the air mounts—periodically shattered by a resident's inane and inappropriate joke.

"It's like the troops in the trenches," says Lloyd. "They're tossing cracks around because they're shit scared. Personally I become very quiet. That's my nature. The worse the crisis, the quieter I become. You have to be calm if you're captain of the ship."

Listening to the Minitor radios, which all members of the trauma team carry clipped to their waistband, pocket, or belt, everyone knows that the Pittsburgh Medic Ambulance is nearing the hospital. The dispatcher in the Communications Center counts down the ETA, three minutes, two minutes, one minute. Suddenly, two paramedics burst through the ER door, literally running down the hall pushing a stretcher. The child is underneath a mound of blankets, soaked with blood. A nurse yells, "Everyone out of here who doesn't belong. There are too many people in the Trauma Room." A few observers leave. Lloyd slips inside, disappearing as the door slams shut. The little boy died three hours later, despite the trauma team's full-scale effort.

The Benedum Pediatric Trauma Program, although a very positive achievement in terms of saving lives, triggered a difficult transition for the Emergency Room staff when it was initiated in 1984, especially for the nurses, according to head nurse Maureen Cusack, who has worked at Children's Hospital for nearly twenty years. "Previously, the child run over by a tractor would have been put in an ambulance and taken to the closest hospital. Now people are being picked up by the helicopter and brought to this Emergency Room, so we are seeing an increased number of very, very severely injured children. Some of these kids probably did not have a chance, no matter what would have happened after the accident." The upshot, said Cusack, is that "many are dying here instead of at the other hospitals."

The first few months as a designated trauma center was "absolutely devastating, and I reacted in a way that I could not have predicted. I got mean, just downright mean. If we had a death in the ER, and I went home and somebody said, 'My shoes hurt,' I would say, 'You're lucky you have feet.'"

Throughout that entire first year, Cusack sensed the onset of a deep-seated depression among her nurses, and she began to feel within herself a mounting pressure to explode. In fact, she could pinpoint the exact moment when this explosion occurred.

The tragic death of the three-year-old who had been playing at home with his father's .357 magnum, was followed the next day by the death of Moira Whitehead. Moira had been a resident at Children's Hospital, who, during each of the three years of her pediatric training, had labored many months in the ER. It had been Moira's birthday, or her husband's birthday, Maureen could not remember which, and they had gone out to dinner to celebrate. Moira had suddenly said, "I feel dizzy," and slumped over on her husband's shoulder. It was determined that she had suffered a coronary thrombosis, which had caused a fatal heart attack. Moira was the same age as Laurie Penix and Molly O'Gorman, as well as many of Maureen Cusack's nurses.

Three days later, there were two additional deaths in the Emergency Room just a few hours apart. The infant son of a young woman serving a fellowship in the Department of Endocrinology had been napping peacefully at home, but when the babysitter peeked into the bedroom, she discovered the little boy dead, undoubtedly of SIDS (Sudden Infant Death Syndrome). Then a beautiful four-year-old who had been visiting Pittsburgh with her parents from British Columbia was involved in an auto accident. She had been admitted to the hospital through the ER, and she arrested in Trauma Room 1.

Even with the introduction of the trauma program, the saving grace for the nurses had been that most of the worst tragedies in the Emergency Room seemed to occur throughout the summer months. June, July, and August would be terrible, and then, when the kids went back to school, it slowed down. There were bad days from time to time during the winter, especially with the first snow, which brought auto accidents along with concussions, bumps, bruises, broken bones—hazards of sled riding, mostly. The nurses could tolerate these difficult days and nights because they could expect relief afterward—a cushion for recovery.

But for Cusack and her nurses, four deaths in the space of a few days was simply unjust. It was always awful when a child was denied the opportunity to live, but when people she knew, people with whom she'd worked, shared grief and sorrow with, died at the same time, she began to question basic beliefs.

"I usually can distance myself a little bit, or take a walk around the block, and come back and feel . . . not better, but in control. And this time I couldn't," said Cusack, who is short, with reddish-brown hair, and has the very direct manner characteristic of most veteran head nurses. These men and women have learned over the years the importance of facing the truth head-on, not attempting to nurture their own vulnerability.

"I took the four-year-old to the morgue, and she was a beautiful little girl. She had black shiny hair. Her little toenails were painted." The morgue is in the basement of the hospital. When transferred for "posting" (post-mortem/autopsy), the dead child will have been thoroughly washed and groomed, a tiny bundle wrapped in soft blue linen towels.

"The man in the morgue did nothing wrong," said Cusack. He didn't grab the body and throw it on the table. He didn't joke or say anything inappropriate. It was a routine transaction, smooth and businesslike, polite and cordial, but she could feel herself, deep inside, losing control. "I wanted to go for his throat. I just wanted to kill him."

Now she paused to light a cigarette. At Children's Hospital, smoking, even behind closed office doors, is a carefully savored secret. "When you've been nursing as long as I have, you know when you're kind of losing it. So I left the hospital and went across the street to Wendy's for a cup of coffee. Now, you know where the homeless people sit in the front by the window? Well, I sat down there to have coffee, and then they started to play those goddam Christmas carols, and you know what happened?" She paused. "I started to cry."

Every day of her working life, Monday through Friday, she walked by Wendy's in the morning on her way to the hospital, noting with sad amusement the bizarre collection of eccentrics and derelicts who gathered in the front part of the dining area—talking to themselves, singing, shouting, crying. Suddenly she had become, at least for that moment, a member of their little inner sanctum.

"I was one of the homeless people that day," said Maureen Cusack.

Chapter 24

As director of Social Services at Children's Hospital, where she has worked since earning her master's degree at the University of Pittsburgh in 1967, Sue Hughes was well aware of the tragic siege the nurses in the Emergency Room were attempting to weather. The deaths themselves were extraordinarily sad, but Hughes was especially concerned with the emotional and physical toll taken on the ER staff, specifically the nurses.

Physicians are privileged: after the crisis is over, they can leave—whatever the outcome. Even the social workers, as liaisons between the physician and family, have a certain flexibility. But the nurses are embroiled in tragedy through to the bitter end, watching in silence the drama played out by frantic family members. Even when it is finally over, nurses are obligated to clean the body and the blood on the floor, replenish supplies, fill out the paperwork—and then finish their shift.

"This whole aspect of so many deaths in the hospital due to the introduction of both the trauma and the transplantation programs has been something that's worried me for a long time," said Hughes. "I think I told you about the Bereavement Committee. We've started a monthly memorial service for children and their parents, but it is long past the time we should be paying attention to similar problems within our own staff."

In fact, Hughes had no sooner finalized details for those monthly services when she spotted Maureen Cusack returning from Wendy's.

"She looked ghastly," said Hughes, and I said, 'How are you?' " Cusack tried to explain the anxiety she had just experienced, but once again she started to cry.

"I said to her, 'Why don't we get everybody together and just talk about how horrible it's been lately?' So that's what we did. One of the most beneficial things that you can do in these horrible crisis situations is give people an opportunity to ventilate."

The discussion that afternoon went on more than an hour—and even when the nurses had returned to work, they continued to talk among themselves. For days afterward, they aired their bad dreams and their insecurities to one another in the coffee room during their breaks, in the narrow nurses' station adjacent to the OBS rooms, or at Peter's Pub across the street and down the block, where the ER nurses sometimes gather after their shifts.

"People said a lot of things that were very healthy to get out into the open," said Cusack. They discovered that they were looking at one another, as well as those loved ones at home, and thinking similar sad and depressing thoughts. "Should I say goodbye to you now?" they asked themselves as they looked around at one another that afternoon. "Am I ever going to see you again?" The nurse working in critical-care situations, says Hughes, is always on the bare edge of negative expectation.

Nurses with children of their own will often be more acutely and personally affected when death occurs in a pediatric institution, says Cusack. "They tell themselves that it could have been their own child. They intimately identify more with the mother's grief, and think, 'I would die if this happened to me.' " This is an especially difficult occurrence for a nurse who is pregnant because it casts a gruesome shadow of uncertainty over the image of beauty and perfection that she is visualizing for her own future.

The younger nurses will also grieve deeply—but differently. "With that four-year-old British Columbia kid," said Cusack, "I found one of the very newest nurses in one of the trauma rooms crying, just crying, and she said, 'I don't know why. I don't know why I'm crying.' That's what she said."

This confusion is understandable and predictable, says Rita Harrison, who works as a psychiatric nurse counselor at Children's. "When you're twenty-two, you are not as well defended against life's stresses. Your skin gets a little thicker as you get older, and you learn ways to put distance between yourself and things that bother you. Part of what's nice about being twenty-two is that everything is fresh, but the flip side of that is that you're not as well protected. When people talk about losing the innocence of their youth, they are not talking about experiences, they're talking about attitude, and a feeling about things not being fresh anymore."

A head nurse, who often serves as a role model and mother figure, must be tender and attentive to younger nurses, usually recent graduates, experiencing a patient's death for the first time. This is an initiation, a passage through which all nurses who work in a tense and highly demanding environment must travel—a sad and unavoidable voyage that remains forever in the nurse's consciousness.

"This happened to a new nurse, twenty-one years old, just yesterday," says Beverly Sahlaney, head nurse of both the Neonatal Intensive Care Unit (NICU) and the Respiratory Care Unit (RCU) at Children's, which, along with the ER and the ICU, are classified as critical-care facilities. "I went to be with her right away, even before the baby was dead," when it was clear that death was imminent. "I knew that the baby was taken care of, we had other nurses covering that baby at that time. The social worker and another nurse were with the mom and dad. So I went to be with that young nurse, who probably needed me more than anybody else did. I asked her, 'Do you want to continue to take care of this baby, or would you like me to change assignments?'

"And she didn't say anything, and then I said, 'I really think it would be better for you if you took care of this baby.'

"Because she needed to know that she could live with herself, she needed to know in the days to come that she could go through the whole process. And she did. She was in tears, but she returned to the bedside, and she picked up the baby and held it.

"And after the baby died, she picked it up again and held it close to her. She held the baby because Mom and Dad could not hold the baby. Mom wanted to remember the baby the way he was when he was not sick.

"So holding that baby served several purposes: Mom and Dad wanted somebody to hold that baby, but they did not want to themselves, and so she helped the family by doing that. But she also helped herself, because she was able to go through the whole process with this little baby, and with this family. And after the baby died, she carried him downstairs to the morgue, where he was going to have his autopsy.

"So she went through all the sequences: The care of this baby, then the baby's dying, and finally the baby's death. And I think that the right decision was made, for her to continue with that baby, but for her also to take note—to know in her heart—that she had someone to talk to, someone to be with her at all times. Because you need to know you are not going through this alone. That's too hard.

"You see, this has happened to me. I've been that nurse taking care of the baby at times, and the baby has died, and I learned that the best thing was to do all you could for the baby, and for the family, extend yourself to the maximum, because in the end you have to live with yourself."

Weeks later, I met Darla Pilarsky, the nurse whose story Sahlaney told.

"It was the first time I had really dealt with anybody, professionally or personally, who was dying," said Pilarsky. "But that day I came in to work overtime, because they needed help, and they assigned me to take care of Adam. About two hours after I started, they did his EEG, and everything was flat and nonreactive, and the parents decided that they were going to withdraw support. Right then and there, I just got a knot in my stomach, because I knew that this was my first time. 'Don't cry, don't do anything'—it was like I was really trying to talk myself into holding back from feeling anything. And then the parents didn't want to hold him, and as bad as I felt, and as teary-eyed as I was, I decided I wanted to hold him, somebody had to hold him. I just felt it was unfair to allow him to die alone.

"Since then, I've gone through this experience two or three more times. And it gets easier, not so much easier emotionally, but you're in better control of it. You might only cry one or two tears instead of sitting there bawling your eyes out. It's not as gut-wrenching as it is the first time. You keep wiping your eyes, but it's easier to hold back. It never feels better—it's just easier to hold back until you're driving home by yourself and nobody can see you crying."

Just as in most other professions, there are styles and philosophies in pediatric nursing that vary a great deal from head nurse to head nurse and, subsequently, from unit to unit. Beverly Sahlaney believes in complete and total involvement of the nurse with the child for which she is caring—a belief she has practiced since her first days at Children's Hospital fifteen years ago. In contrast, Kathy Nelson, a former head nurse in the oncology unit at Children's, today a clinical nurse specialist (master's degree) in oncology, contends that this intense style of care is harmful to the nurse as well as the patient. "I'll find nurses coming in on their days off to visit a family; they'll bring presents for the kids—not all the kids, just certain kids. I had a staff nurse take a parent home to sleep in her house, that sort of thing. To me, that's overinvolvement. At that point they've crossed over the line and have become a friend, a part of the family, and consequently cannot function at a therapeutic level."

Sahlaney disagrees, believing that a nurse's intense involvement enhances her effectiveness. "If you can get emotionally involved in that baby and that family, then you're going to treat that baby as though he's yours, and you're going to have the utmost respect for that baby, and you're going to make sure your hands are cleaner, and you're going to make sure you go home and read a little bit about that disease. The closer you get to that family, the more you put into the care of that child. And the more you put into the care of that child, the longer he remains with us. So I will cross the line," says Sahlaney. "I will not pull back."

Although their philosophies about nursing disagree, I discovered that there are only minor differences in the way in which Sahlaney and Nelson approach their patients.

"What's happening with Marco?" asks Nelson one morning, beginning her rounds at Children's on Unit 8 North.

"He don't look so good today," his mother answers.

Marco, six years old, is slender and emaciated, his skin almost translucent in its paleness. Underneath his bright red baseball cap he is completely bald, having lost his hair during chemotherapy.

"He used to get up in the morning and eat a half gallon of ice cream," the mother says. "Now he don't even like ice cream no more. All he eats is chicken. I made him eat five legs of chicken last night, and today, I got chicken for his lunch. We're going to chicken that kid to death."

Marco has been taking chemotherapy through the veins in his wrist, but soon he is going to require an entryway into his torso, Nelson explains. There are two choices: You can use a Broviac Catheter, a tiny tube that is implanted, hanging loosely two inches down the chest, or a port, which, because it is implanted flush against the chest, is less visible, but "there's a little pinch when the needle goes in."

A boy named John, who has been playing with a little red-and-white plastic robot, stands up to show me his port. He pulls up his striped jersey and exhibits it proudly, then returns to the toy, which he is systematically dismantling with a plastic hammer. John and Marco are laughing and pushing one another playfully. Suddenly, a woman enters the room. It's John's mother.

"John, Sally wants you. She's ready."

Abruptly, John drops the hammer, turns on his heels, and stomps determinedly down the hall. He walks into the room in which he will receive his chemotherapy. The door closes. A deafening silence fills the air, shattered by a piercing wail of fear.

Although cancer is one of the dirtiest words in America, Nelson stresses that cancer in children is different from that in adults. "I think we have more hope for children, particularly those with leukemia and with Wilms' tumor [which occurs in the kidney]. Today we have a very good outlook for kids with Hodgkin's disease as well. We've made a lot of progress."

She does not attribute the progress in helping to cure cancer only to science, however. Nelson credits the special spirit of children for much of the success. "They don't sit in the corner and mope very much. Most of them, especially the little ones, have a strong drive to grow and develop and play and keep on fighting, despite the pain. I tell the parents right from the beginning, 'You're going to get your inspiration from seeing this youngster get better.' That's the plus side of working with kids. Some do get depressed, have their down times and their sick times, but they possess a special and unconscious drive to grow and get well."

Although some of her children will not survive the treatment intended to cure them, Nelson believes that John and Marco will. She introduces me to four-year-old Jason, who has already survived the worst of his treatment. "He's in remission."

Since he is being released from the hospital tomorrow, the discussion with his mother focuses upon Jason's followup treatment, his return visits. Oblivious to the proceedings, Jason busies himself by acting out the story of his young life. He goes into the bathroom, closes the door, knocks on the door, opens it, comes out, and closes the door. Then he knocks on the door, repeating the process, back and forth, opening and closing the door. "I'm home and I'm here," he says to Nelson. "I'm here, I'm home, I'm here."

After visiting fourteen patients in various stages of recovery or relapse through the morning, we stop to see nineteen-year-old Marissa, who has decided that her Broviac is too visible and bothersome. She wants a port. The surgeon who is going to do this procedure has directed Nelson to meet with Marissa and put an X with a ballpoint pen on the exact spot on her chest where the entry-way should be placed.

Marissa doesn't want it too close to her breasts, she says. And she doesn't want it up so high on her chest that people can easily see it. A long conversation ensues between her eighteen-year-old husband and her mother, but as soon as they begin speaking, Marissa turns in the opposite direction and stares idly at the TV. Most of Nelson's long-time patients react similarly. They listen, they nod, they smile, and they shrug. Eventually, they grit their teeth and go forward with whatever therapy is necessary, hoping that it will end eventually, one way or the other, just as wakefulness does at the conclusion of each day.

When her rounds are completed, Nelson explains that Children's Hospital remains loyal to all its pediatric oncology patients, even if they pass the hospital's eighteen-year-old age limit, like Marissa. "They can always come back to Children's. They don't have to change the continuity of their care, even if they are in their thirties. As long as they live, they can return here. My kids don't leave me," Nelson adds, "unless—or until—until they die."

Part V

Intensive Care

Chapter 25

A PEDIATRIC intensivist is a physician whose primary specialty is pediatrics with a subspecialty in the newly created field of critical care. The field is so new, in fact, that in 1988 the first national examination for pediatric critical care certified only two hundred intensivists to serve in the six hundred pediatric intensive-care units listed with the American Hospital Association.

Anesthesiology is the field from which many intensivists come, because the basic skills of critical-care medicine—inserting a tube into the trachea and connecting that tube to a ventilator, for instance—are skills that are also mastered by the anesthesiologist. Critical care actually fell under the anesthesiologists' umbrella by default: Surgeons and internists had too many other pressing responsibilities for them to keep a constant vigil on unstable patients once a case in the OR was completed, but the anesthesiologist was more flexible.

Florence Nightingale first began the practice of concentrating critically ill patients in one predesignated area 140 years ago. In 1952, during the polio epidemic in Copenhagen, medical students were drafted in order to do tracheostomies on paralyzed patients who were unable to breathe. But the concept of a central intensive-care center was not wholeheartedly adopted until 1958, when Peter Safar, then at Johns Hopkins University, the man who was to prove the validity of mouth-to-mouth resuscitation and later CPR (cardiopulmonary resuscitation), established the first adult intensive-care unit in the world. Safar moved his operations to Pittsburgh a few years later, developing a state-of-the-art ICU at Presbyterian-University Hospital, and Children's Hospital followed soon after with a pediatric unit. Safar had a great interest in helping to establish a pediatric ICU, for he was convinced that a pediatric intensivist might have saved his child, who died in the early 1960s.

Prior to that time, anesthesiologists stabilized especially critical patients in the recovery room and subsequently in corridors, storerooms—any nook or cranny with close proximity to the operating room. Situated in a ward or private room four or five floors away from the primary physician, the patient was especially vulnerable, despite a nurse's careful attention.

With the rapid increase in intensive-care units in hospitals across the United States, and the addition of ICUs designated for other specialties—such as cardiology, neurology, and burn units—the intensivists began to assert their independence. They contended that the challenges in the ICU—the intricate technology, the reactions and complications of high-risk surgery, such as organ transplantation, and the vulnerability of these patients to a myriad of esoteric infections—sufficiently separated the critical-care specialist from any other field.

Because of the nature of critical care, intensivists are an idiosyncratic and generally isolated breed. Whereas the surgeon, the cardiologist, the endocrinologist, or the specialist in infectious disease will regularly round throughout the hospital, the intensivist while on duty is essentially confined within the walls of the unit.

The forty-three beds in the ICU, Neonatal Intensive Care Unit (NICU), and Respiratory Care Unit (RCU) at Children's Hospital are all supervised by medical director Ann Thompson, who is assisted by four other ICU attendings, who have joint appointments in the Department of Pediatrics at Pitt. Approximately eight fellows in the unit have completed three-year residencies in pediatrics, undergoing Children's three-year subspecialty training program in pediatric intensive care.

In addition to the fellows, there are pediatric residents, as well as attendings, residents, and nurse coordinators from other specialties and subspecialties (transplantation, cardiology, ENT, etc.), whose patients are being treated in the ICU. There are physical therapists and respiratory therapists. There is a child life specialist. There are clergy, and there is a social worker to deal with the family—which is, of course, on the scene on a regular basis—parents and grandparents included. In contrast to the stark reality of what it means to be admitted to the ICU—the patient must be critically ill—it is a bright, highly populated, sometimes noisy arena.

Thompson, who five years ago, at thirty-five, became one of the youngest ICU medical directors in the nation, shoulders overall responsibility for the unit, assisted by four attendings, who are associate medical directors. Each of the five (including Thompson) assumes hands-on control of the unit on a rotating basis for one week. Subsequent weeks are left free to help in the unit, write papers, launch research projects and follow through on them, and satisfy administrative responsibilities. "One week" does not mean eight hours, Monday through Friday, or even twelve hours; it means that the attending will be in the unit or immediately available to it unfailingly throughout a six-day, 144-hour period. Sleeping at home most of those nights is possible but not to be expected; returning to the unit in the early morning hours for an emergency situation is routine.

The week "on call" for the attending begins on Friday with Monday as an off day, then continues Tuesday through Thursday. Fellows assume an even more rigorous schedule, sharing night call once every four nights in addition to their regular daily routine. Depending on other demands upon ICU physicians, such as transport and trauma team responsibilities, there will be three or four fellows in the unit at any one time through the morning, afternoon, and early evening, and one or two fellows at night.

"At the end of a shift, you feel pretty 'grody,' " says Denise Goodman, an ICU fellow in her third year of training. "You find yourself shrinking from humanity as the day goes on. Morning starts, the afternoon, the night; the next morning—and you have the same clothes on. You've been so busy, you haven't brushed your teeth, and you've only been to the john twice in twenty-four hours. People don't want to stand next to you. They turn away when you try to talk."

Throughout the day, there is an underlying subdued commotion that pervades the brightly lighted atmosphere of the ICU. The equipment attached to each patient in this age of technology is confounding. To name only a small part of the technology readily available, there are ventilators, to breathe for patients or to help them breathe; cardiac output machines, to measure the exact amount of blood that the heart pumps per beat; heart-lung machines, often referred to as "pumps"; electrocardiographs, to perform electrocardiograms (EKGs), a diagnostic test that records the electric activity of the heart in a wave-form pattern; electroencephalographs (EEGs), to record brain activity; and oxygen-saturation monitors, also called pulse oximeters, electronic devices that attach to the patient's forefinger, seeming to make the finger glow, to simultaneously monitor pulse rate and percentage of oxygen in the patient's blood. There are television monitors, tangles of lines, tubes, and catheters. There is a constant cacophony of alarms and buzzers.

Three Extra Corporeal Membrane Oxygenation (ECMO) units usually operate simultaneously in the ICU—a passive support system for newborn babies with weakened, irritated, or infected lungs. ECMO, pioneered at Children's Hospital and a few other centers, provides babies with an artificial lung in combination with cardiopulmonary bypass—it pumps blood through the circulatory system as would the healthy heart—to keep a baby alive until the lungs are mature enough to handle the breathing process independently. Only patients with at least a 20 percent likelihood of survival are normally put on ECMO, 80 percent of whom do survive. Children's Hospital is one of the largest and busiest ECMO centers in the United States, saving lives at a rate of three infants a month.

Since many of the patients in the ICU are comatose and all are extraordinarily sick, most are given blood, nutrition, and medication through lines, the most common of which is an intravenous infusion. There are also A lines, or arterial lines, useful for patients with respiratory difficulties or for frequent monitoring of arterial blood gases. A lines are also the most accurate and direct means of measuring blood pressure. There are femoral or radial artery lines, pulmonary artery lines, and CVPs (central venous pressure) lines used to deliver fluids or medications to measure vascular pressures within the heart. Because children have such tiny veins and arteries, and because a needle must be inserted precisely and directly into them in order for lines to function effectively, sinking, or starting, lines can be frustrating, tedious, and, unfortunately, incredibly bloody.

Former ICU fellow Steve Lawless, today an attending at the University of North Carolina, says that he is often amazed that the people involved in critical care can handle the stress. "I just find it absolutely mind-boggling that I can do it, or the nurses, or the respiratory therapists, day in and day out. Hearing the monitors go off, the alarms and beeps—all that noise. At home after a shift, it sometimes takes me an hour in my bed to settle down." A visitor to the unit can easily understand the phrase "ICU psychosis," used to describe the long-term patient's confusion—a lack of awareness about time and place, a loss of a sense of self.

The ICU is the hub of the hospital, through which most major services rotate, often sharing responsibility for a patient. "It could be a multiple-trauma kid who has a head injury, a busted leg, and an abdominal laceration," according to attending intensivist Pat Kochanek. "You've got the general surgeons, the orthopedic surgeons, the neurosurgeons, the ICU team, and an array of other specialties descending upon the kid at the same time—and often disagreeing about the approach to treatment."

When such disagreements occur, the attending specialist maintains authority over his or her area of expertise while the intensivist both mediates and analyzes to make sure that a recommended intervention—invasive or noninvasive (such as medication)—although therapeutic on one level, will not be harmful to another area of the body. The intensivist must liaison with and support all specialists, subspecialists, technicians, and supplemental staff—with the overall well-being and ultimate survival of the patient as his or her primary responsibility.

Intensivists find a special joy and challenge in working under pressure, according to intensivist Brad Fuhrman. "Most pediatricians have a limited number of procedures that they do on a regular basis. They may start IVs, do spinal taps, or suture in the ER, but with the procedures we get to do in intensive care, our backs are often against the wall: establishing an airway when someone can't breathe, or putting in a central catheter to restore blood volume in someone who is in shock. These things carry a certain amount of adrenaline with them, but they are also very therapeutic. That is, right there at bedside, you can do something that will make the difference between living and dying."

Intensivists are action-oriented individuals, trained to respond instinctively and immediately in crisis situations. "You can walk into the unit in the morning, and it is pretty relaxed, ten or fifteen kids, most of them on the mend," says Denise Goodman. "Two hours later, it's mass bedlam, twenty-five patients, two crashes [emergencies], one on either corner of the unit. So you run here trying to plug your finger in the dike, run there, plug your finger in a different dike, get a phone call, 'Denise, we need another bed for an incoming transplant patient,' get called to a floor for an arrest, and all of a sudden, your beeper goes off: 'Transport physician—incoming call—you are needed on the heliopad posthaste,' or 'Trauma Physician—Level I trauma, head injury, massive bleeding en route to the ER, ETA five minutes.'

"People sometimes think that I am a high-key person because I am constantly talking aloud to myself and making lists. But you have to stratify responsibilities in your own mind consciously and regularly: 'Okay, I have these ten things to do, what's the most important? Second most important, third? What can wait until tomorrow, the next day, the day after?' In the ICU, your priorities are always changing—sometimes by the minute."

A major frustration for the intensivist, according to Ann Thompson, is that most people, even in the medical world, do not precisely understand what the intensivist does. "If someone says, 'What does a surgeon do?', you can point to a procedure that fixed something, and that's really very understandable and satisfying. If you're a cardiologist, you figure out what's wrong with somebody's heart, and then you provide them with medication until it is time for a cardiac surgeon to fix it. The pulmonologist looks at the lungs, the nephrologist looks at the kidneys, the neurologist looks at the brain. They tend to focus upon diseases that live in one place.

"But we sit in some kind of never-never land between the specialties, focusing on the interaction between the systems. We attempt to support one system without damaging another."

Unfortunately for the intensivist, when the patient recovers, as most patients do, they will usually be much more grateful to the surgeons, if a procedure was required, or to the nurses and doctors who cared for them after ICU when they were conscious enough to be aware of names, voices, and faces. (Patients are often paralyzed in the ICU—medicated—in order to pass more calmly through crisis situations.) "Kids will occasionally come back and visit, but it doesn't happen very often," Fuhrman says.

In contrast to virtually every other unit in the hospital, where nurses are assigned responsibility for anywhere from four to six patients, ostensibly in separate rooms, nurses in a pediatric ICU must be situated at a patient's bedside, or between two patients at most, keeping constant vigil. One-on-one in the ICU is even more imperative in pediatrics because children are harder to reason with than adults, according to ICU head nurse Tammy Fleeger. "You tell an adult, 'Don't shake your head back and forth, because that tube that is helping you breathe will come out,' and an adult will understand and comply with your request. All a kid knows is that he hates this thing in his throat and he's going to thrash until he gets rid of it. That's why the constant surveillance is essential."

A nurse's work schedule revolves around the times to take vital signs. "That's when you usually do a good assessment, do other routine things, such as chest physiotherapy and suctioning; most of the kids in our unit are here for pulmonary care. And then you have your schedule of medications that you work around. IV tubings and pressure tubings get changed every day. It's not a major thing, if you're experienced, but it does take a certain amount of time.

"The prioritization takes place when something happens that is not scheduled. Something in your child's status changes—he's getting sicker and sicker, crashing. Or more simply, you find that you need to take your patient off the unit for a CT [computerized tomography] scan. If it's a kid you can sit in a wheelchair and push, well, that's not much of a deal. But for our patients, you have to take them to CT on the bed, and you have to find a way to move them in this bed with all their IV pumps, all their equipment attached. You have to have some way for them to breathe while you get them there, because they are on a ventilator (a respiratory therapist must come along), so it can take an hour out of your day."

Nursing in the ICU is an intensely focused experience; complete concentration is essential. "When I first walked into this unit," says RN Rita Harrison, a counselor for critical-care nurses under stress, "I remember thinking how profoundly grateful I was that I don't do pediatric nursing. In adult critical care, we have some small margin for error, more than people realize, but in pediatric critical care, you have none at all.

"Just for an example, if you give an adult patient 100 ccs of fluid, more or less, it's very rarely going to make a difference. But with a child, you would never even give that much at any one time. There is absolutely no room for any kind of human error. It's very daunting to realize that someone must work for a twelve-hour span in a situation where the normal propensity to err even a little bit can be so critical."

Counting pediatric ICU, RCU, and NICU combined, there are about 125 nurses working critical care at Children's Hospital, mostly on twelve-hour shifts, seven days every two weeks. Many of those days off are consumed by emergency overtime, however. The average pediatric critical-care nurse will burn out and eventually leave the unit within 2.1 years—a little more than six months longer than it takes to train them. On the average, according to an editorial in *Nursing Times,* "nurses at the age of 45 can expect to live another 26.9 years, about two years less than people in comparable professions."

Tammy Fleeger's assistant head nurse, David Silay, one of the five male critical-care nurses working at Children's full-time, observes few differences in the way in which nurses of opposite sexes respond to crisis or tragedy, but he does acknowledge a significant contrast in how his women colleagues deal with the business-oriented side of their profession.

Traditionally, says Silay, nurses have had a tendency to transfer to other hospitals every few years and not worry too much about matters such as length of tenure and retirement benefits, figuring that "others—husbands—would take care of them." But times are different. Nurses must learn to be much more hardheaded and practical. "I've said point-blank to a lot of nurses in meetings, 'There's no guarantee that you're ever going to get married; you really better start thinking about life down the road and being on your own.'"

Patty Schaal, a psychologist who, along with Rita Harrison, provides psychiatric counseling at Children's, agrees with Silay, pointing out that public school teachers made few financial inroads until men began to infiltrate the profession. In 1988, the Pittsburgh Federation of Teachers signed a contract with the Pittsburgh Board of Education establishing a maximum annual salary for teachers with a minimum of eight years' service of $52,000—for nine and a half months of teaching. The maximum annual salary for comparable years of service at Children's Hospital and at most other health-care institutions in the state of Pennsylvania ranges between $30,000 and $35,000, with three weeks of vacation annually.

Men are only now beginning to look seriously at nursing as a profession, for it is not easy or socially acceptable in some quarters for a man to be a nurse, says Schaal, whose husband teaches nursing on the university level. "He has a doctorate, and people say, 'Oh, Dr. Schaal. What do you teach?' And after all these years, I still hear him. There's a hesitancy before he can say, 'I teach nursing.'"

Chapter 26

THE Respiratory Care Unit (RCU) in which Danielle Burdette has lived most of her life is designed primarily for chronically (although not acutely) ill patients who require constant monitoring and regular nursing attention. Because of their reliance on the ventilator, the children in RCU cannot be sent to the other units of the hospital, and because of the expense, many cannot be cared for at home, where round-the-clock nursing would be essential. According to head nurse Beverly Sahlaney, "One little girl, three years old, has Werdnig-Hoffmann disease [a progressive, genetic neuromuscular disease]. She's not able to move her hands or feet. Even when she is crying or smiling, it's hard actually to see what she's doing—except that when she's crying you will see little tears coming down her cheeks. The little girl next to her, her younger sister, has the same problem."

The sisters cannot recover, Sahlaney explained, "but they could go home with the right home environment, with twenty-four-hour nursing care. But until the time comes when Mom and Dad feel that they are ready to take these two little girls home, they need to be cared for somewhere, and right now Children's Hospital's RCU is the place." Although there are a number of nursing homes for adults with similar chronic conditions, there are very few facilities willing or able to care for the ventilated chronically ill child.

At a certain point, the parents, fully informed of the condition of their children at birth, had the option of terminating the use of the ventilator, ending the child's life. "We talked to them before the second child was actually ventilated, because we knew what kind of course this child was going to have, based upon the older sister. 'If we put this child on a ventilator, she will then live. Do you want to go through that?' And they decided, yes, they did; they wanted to go through the same course with the younger sister."

Sahlaney says that initially the parents of these two girls were quite dedicated, but over time they have become less attentive. "There are other children at home. They have work, they have obligations, and after weeks, and months, and years, it's almost a protection. They don't want to bond with the child because they are afraid they are going to lose her. They go back and forth. They stay away for a long time, then they might come in for a couple of days in a row. It's very difficult to have a child that's not normal when, looking at the world around you, there are so many people who are vibrant, and interested in life. This mom can see a little three-year-old child walking down the street, laughing and skipping, eating an ice cream cone, knowing her child can't do that."

Sahlaney explains that the nurses try to establish a comfortable and nonthreatening environment for the children in RCU. "We want to give those children not only the physical care but also the developmental care, the socialization that they would get outside. In the daytime, they need to get out of their pajamas, get into regular clothes; they need to get out of their beds. If you go there in the daytime, and it's not nap period, most of the kids will be in a high chair, in a walker, in a stroller, in a chair. They do not belong in bed in the daytime. If they were at home, Mom wouldn't have them in bed all day, and we want to be as close to a home-type environment as we can and still be within the walls of a hospital."

Part of the day, children who are ventilated and/or paralyzed or comatose lie on mattresses on the floor so that parents and nurses can play and relate more directly with them, at their own level. In addition to the normal sounds of the unit, the regular thumping of the ventilators, the beeping of alarms, the conversations between nurses, parents, and physicians, distant voices can constantly be heard in the background—not real conversation, but soothing sounds from tape recorders lying on pillows alongside a child's ear. The children are listening to the voices of mothers or fathers who cannot, for one reason or another, be with them.

"We have moms and dads and siblings talk, sing, or read stories on tapes, and then send them to us, and then we play them for the baby. We had one mom who was here for a good while but needed to return to Philadelphia to care for other children. A week or two later, she came back to see her little baby and she was so upset because he kept looking away from her, to the left. When she told me that, I realized what was happening. We always put the tape recorder to his left, so he was responding to her voice by looking in that direction.

"She was a good mom; she brought tapes that had Bible stories, and she would be reading a Bible story to the baby, and then she'd stop the story, and say, 'Now, Christopher, it is a real nice day out today, the sun is shining,' and she'd just go on, talking to Christopher, and then she'd go back to the story, and read some more of the story, and then she'd stop and talk to Christopher again. And you knew it had an impact on that baby, if he reacted to her voice in person like he did to the tape."

Later, Sahlaney led me into the RCU and introduced me to Shirley Austin, who was waiting in the unit with her daughter, Nikki, for release the following day. Sahlaney explained that Nikki had been ill with spina bifida, but that after a long stay at Children's she had been doing well on home ventilator care until she had contracted a sudden virus, which brought her back to the hospital. Nikki had weathered the crisis, but she was not the same child that she was before she became infected. The virus had so severely damaged her brain that the parents had decided to put her on DNR status, Do Not Resuscitate. And although the parents were taking their child home tomorrow, they realized that she no longer had much personality or spirit.

Shirley Austin was a woman in shock. When she began relating her thoughts and fears it was as if she had suddenly exploded, and desperately needed to tell it to somebody, anybody, who would listen and perhaps understand at least part of it. She told me about how her husband, Jeffrey, hated hospitals and how he had initially refused to come in, even to see Nikki, whom he deeply loved. And how every time he forced himself to walk into the RCU, he began to cry because of the suffering that the babies—his and all the others—had to endure. She told me about how you get involved with the problems of other people and their children. She pointed across the room to a tiny black girl lying in bed and said, "Brain tumor." She motioned at the parents. "Two weeks ago, they had a healthy child on their hands. Now they're waiting for her to be dead." She pointed to the bed where Danielle Burdette lay. "I couldn't conceive of going through what that woman has endured throughout the life of her child."

Shirley Austin told me that $300,000 of the maximum of $500,000 of her medical insurance had already been eaten up. The cost of each day in RCU is equal to more than a week of what it would cost her at home, even with twenty-four-hour-a-day nursing care. She said that when Nikki begins to have breathing problems, the alarm to the ventilator might not go off. And so, although she could skimp and save by not having a night nurse for the eight hours in which the child would normally sleep, she would never feel completely confident that her child would be alive the following morning. Nikki looked very pink and healthy—pudgy, with big, round blue eyes. I reached out and stroked her arm. She was as warm and soft as any other baby, but forever different.

All patients in the RCU and most patients in the ICU are attached to a mechanical apparatus that either partially or totally supports their breathing: a ventilator—a complicated and imposing instrument that controls the number of breaths a patient will take per minute and the ratio of air and oxygen within each inspiration. There are other significant adjustments for patients experiencing especially difficult breathing problems. Referred to as PIP and PEEP, acronyms for "positive inspiratory pressure" and "positive end expiratory pressure," these adjustments are often required to expand weakened alveola, the tiny structures inside the lungs where the actual exchange of oxygen and carbon dioxide takes place. As patients heal, they will be weaned away from the security of the ventilator, with the number of breaths and the amount of oxygen gradually reduced. After doctor's orders are written, the therapist will assume responsibility for maintaining and calibrating each machine.

Respiratory therapists also serve on the Level I Trauma Team, the Transport Team, and the ECMO units, and regularly respond to Condition A (cardiac arrest) alerts. Although the ICU doctors actually perform the intubation, as well as determine the extent of ventilator support, respiratory therapists, three of whom are on duty full-time in the ICU, are responsible for supplying the vital data upon which the doctors' decisions are based.

In the laboratory across the hall from the ICU, respiratory therapists also rush—on demand and on the spot—blood samples through a process that determines the blood gases, including the pH (the degree of acidity) and the levels of oxygen and carbon dioxide. Whenever certain kinds of diseases occur, primarily respiratory difficulties, blood gases instantaneously provide important diagnostic information. For patients who are critically ill, blood gases are measured frequently, often directly before and after a therapeutic treatment. With the exception of the lab in the ER, respiratory therapists process blood for the entire hospital.

According to Cheryl Krause, who has been a pediatric respiratory therapist at Children's for nine years, the fifty-three employees in the Respiratory Department will spend as much time at the patient's bedside and become as emotionally entangled as any nurse or doctor in the unit.

"We've seen a lot of really nasty stuff, but probably the worst I've ever seen was a family that were in their car and were hit by a coal truck. The mother was killed instantly, the father, who survived with minor injuries, was sent to Presby [Presbyterian-University Hospital] to be treated, the son was transferred to Children's with a broken leg and a few cuts and bruises. And then there were two little girls—the rest of the family—that were brought into the ICU. One was seven and one was five. They had massive head injuries, and they were lying right next to each other." Although the doctors and therapists were able to maintain their vital signs mechanically, the entire ICU staff knew, as they stood vigil over the children through the night, that survival was not possible.

"All night, we had to keep those children alive and breathing. All night long, all we did was pump blood, do gases, push drugs. And all night I cried. I was in that bathroom crying every chance I could get. I think everybody in that unit was devastated, because there were two beautiful little girls, and we had to stand there and watch them." The little girls' conditions were stabilized until the father could recover enough to make some of the necessary decisions. "We had to stand there and watch the father come in. His wife was dead. His son was upstairs, and both his girls were lying there dying. It was awful." The father donated his daughters' organs for transplantation. "So we had to keep them alive even longer, in order to take them to the OR and have the organs removed. It was nightmarish."

Respiratory therapists put in long hours, endure similar emotional trauma, and yet, according to Krause, like the comedian Rodney Dangerfield, they get no respect. Krause and her colleagues do not think that this fact of their lives is very amusing, however.

"We go to school just as long as a nurse does, sometimes longer. We have college degrees [master's degrees are possible], and we have to be registered, just like a nurse." But people both inside and outside the hospital don't understand who they are and why they are there.

She remembers pulling a humidifier up to a child that had been extubated (to clear bronchial passages), "and her mother looked up and smiled and said, 'Well, here's the water girl.' I was extremely offended," says Krause. "I know they're not trying to be mean, but they just don't know."

Chapter 27

LUCKILY, morale is not a particularly serious problem within the confines of Children's Hospital, but it is a fact that many people other than surgeons, pediatricians, nurses, and social workers contribute to the well-being of the institution—including one of the best-equipped and most highly trained private police forces in the western half of the state. In fact, Children's Hospital may be one of the few pediatric institutions guarded by armed officers (twenty-eight at full complement) who are commissioned to make arrests, issue traffic citations, run license plates through the state computer system—virtually any normal law enforcement procedure.

The rationale behind the formation of the Department of Public Safety, according to its director, William Hilf, "is to be absolutely certain that no malicious harm would ever come to the children entrusted to the hospital for care and treatment." As to the .38-caliber weapons his officers carry, a special FBI-approved ammunition was designed by consultants working under his direction, based on research that showed that 99 percent of all firing occurred within 21 feet of the individuals involved. The Children's Hospital bullet is lethal and effective to a maximum of 35 feet. "Beyond that range it just sort of tapers off. If I was to shoot at you and miss, it would hit the wall and nearly crumble. It won't penetrate the wall." Among other duties, including traffic control, officers of the Department of Public Safety answer 150 telephone inquiries and complaints a day, and oversee 250 helicopter landings, answer 900 requests to unlock doors, and conduct 385 escorts each month.

Disorderly conduct and trespassing are the two primary violations resulting in arrest. "We have a lot of family disputes; husbands, boyfriends, come in at different hours"—many unwanted by the women and children they have come to see.

As we walk the corridors of the hospital, twenty-three-year-old Sergeant David Shaulis is not necessarily looking for smokers, but he's going to tag them if he sees them, he says. New city ordinances for public buildings provide fines of $52.50 for a first offense, $100 for a second offense, and up to $300 for a third offense. We start on the top floor and walk each wing, descending from floor to floor. When we reach six, the ICU area, Shaulis says, "My officers don't want to walk through ICU. They say they're afraid they'll set off all the machines with their radios, but I know what the truth is. They don't like to see what's happening here. All the sadness, all the hurt kids, all the frightened families. I try to walk through here every night, however."

We pass the ICU satellite pharmacy, and Shaulis discovers that the alarm hasn't been turned on. With his walkie-talkie, Shaulis calls the command post, summoning someone from the pharmacy downstairs to secure the alarm.

"This is a junkie's candy store," Shaulis says.

Shaulis is proud of the fact that he's the youngest officer in the Department of Public Safety, supervisor of the evening shift. His father, grandfather, and great-grandfather were Pittsburgh policemen.

Recently, he captured an ex-patient who came into the facility with a gun seeking one of the doctors. He talks about staking out an area for a suspected marijuana smoker, and how all the cameras that they had set up, all the additional security precautions, failed to identify the smoker. He had pretty much given up the search when he was rounding one day "and suddenly smelled the stuff. There was a young lady who worked in medical records. She was waving her arm around trying to wipe away the odor when I walked through the door." He reported her and confiscated the marijuana, and she was fired the next day.

"You realize how important it is to be alert in a place like medical records? The surgeons up in the OR, they call downstairs for someone's chart, and they look up what they need to look up, but if they're not given the right record for any reason, do you realize what trouble it could cause?"

Shaulis rounds through all the different nooks and crannies of the hospital: the heliport, where two Children's Hospital police officers must be stationed at fire hoses each time a helicopter lands; the "on call" floor, where doctors on the house staff (residents) can sleep, eat, and talk in private; the elevator machine room on the very top of the old DeSoto wing; the sub-basement with offices for Engineering, Carpentry, Plumbing, Architecture; the boiler room; the furnace room; the print shop; the laundry. Secret but vital places in a complicated and sophisticated health-care complex like Children's.

Children's Hospital at 11 P.M. is a lonely place. Many children are alone, sitting in their beds, watching TV. I see a little boy, bald from repeated chemotherapy, lying on his back, playing with dolls. So many infants, frightened and shrieking. Parents wandering aimlessly through the halls, exhausted but afraid to sleep. Nurses sitting in chairs behind their stations, cuddling with kids. Moms reading bulletin boards in the playroom. As we walk through the ICU on 6 one more time, parents are waiting in line to use the two pay telephones. Some are pacing nervously, while others curl up on chairs and on the floor in corners, crying. As we walk the hospital, especially ICU, the nurses will smile and say to Shaulis:

"Did we do something wrong again?"

Shaulis shakes his head. "I go through here a couple of times every night, and that's their ongoing question." He is silent for a while as we proceed down the hall. Then he stops and turns, almost as if he is considering the possibility of returning to the unit for more specific information. "Why do they keep asking me that?"

There are three large drawings of dinosaurs on the wall outside of the playroom on 8 North—a very popular area in which many of the inpatients congregate—and Carol Siegel is responsible for bringing the children and the dinosaurs together. Working as a consultant for Children's Hospital after the completion of its patient tower, Siegel rounded through the hospital regularly. Siegel's rounds were not for the sake of science, however, but for art. With a $75,000 budget, she was responsible for selecting and hanging the appropriate posters and illustrations befitting the varied areas—and moods—of the hospital.

For Occupational Therapy/Physical Therapy (OTPT), for instance, primarily for handicapped children, drawings with scenes of physical activities—bicycling, baseball, or hockey—would be distasteful. Many of the children in the hospital are on restricted diets, so illustrations with food, ice cream, or candy also had to be eliminated. Anything with religious or sexual connotation was also inappropriate. Walking through the hospital, interviewing staff about preference and taste, Siegel came to appreciate the diversity in decor required.

She discovered that nurses especially were very preoccupied with and sensitive to visions of death. "I had suggested a series of prints symbolizing changes of the season in a park in Paris—summer, fall, winter, spring. The nurses liked spring and summer but refused to have winter and fall for the parent lounge because of the negativity they represent. I have never looked at a scene of winter or autumn and thought of impending death. But at Children's, things are different." Flowers growing in a park or front lawn are acceptable to nurses, says Siegel, but if they are arranged in a vase, nurses often conjure up funeral-oriented images. They are especially opposed to the use of gladiolus, which some nurses maintained were "funeral flowers."

The nurses on the 9th Floor, which is the transplant unit, were easier to get along with, simply because they were willing to accept any artistic creation as long as it did not have as a featured element the color yellow. "Almost everything these nurses deal with on a day-to-day basis is yellow," Siegel explains. "The babies are yellow [jaundiced], everything they throw up is yellow, everything that comes out of their body is yellow. They said, 'We want pink, blue, purple, but nothing yellow.' "

Art selected for the recovery and radiology rooms "focused on the fact that all these kids are in a horizontal position, lying down, almost the whole time they're in there. So they have to be looking up at something. And many have blurred vision because they are just coming out of anesthesia. So the things I suggested were crisp, clear-cut images. Nothing muted, nothing softened, nothing abstracted. Large-scale images that could be immediately recognized, and also at the same time be friendly and comforting." Siegel chose puppies, ducks, colorful wind socks, and kinetic sculptures suspended from the ceiling.

"For 8 North, oncology, that's home to a lot of kids. They are living there until they die. When we were making the presentation to the

Committee [which must approve each illustration before purchase], I was outside the playroom, holding up two posters of dinosaurs— Brontosaurus and Stegosaurus—done in real bright pink and orange and royal and kelly, when a little child came by. She was being pushed in one of those carts with the legs straight out, a pale little thing with an IV in each arm. The child was completely bald, big eyes, and as I'm holding up these two posters, she says, 'Ahhhh. Brontosaurus and Stegosaurus.' This little voice—so excited.

"So I said, 'That's right. Do you like them?'

"She said, 'I love dinosaurs. I love Brontosaurus and Stegosaurus.'

"Then the nurse that was pushing her said, 'Leah, we're going to have these pictures here, and you're going to be able to see them every day.'

"And she said, 'Oh, are we really? Isn't that exciting! Can I go tell my mom?'

"So the Committee said, 'Well, I guess that's a sale. How can we not buy it?' "

The continuous operation of certain basic services, often taken for granted at home or in the office, is much more crucial in a hospital setting, according to William L. Stranahan, Facilities Management and Engineering Services Department assistant manager. Stranahan supervises a staff of fifty-four men and women who, day and night, repair and maintain heating, ventilating, air-conditioning, biomedical, or patient-related electrical equipment. The department maintains more than a million square feet of building, including grounds, parking, sidewalks, patient areas, labs, and departments from the heliport on the roof down to the sub-basement.

Alex Wispolis, director of the Biomedical and Communication Equipment Division and a Children's employee for more than two decades, works directly under Stranahan. Wispolis and his staff are responsible for the calibration, maintenance, and repair of approximately three thousand pieces of medical equipment. "We also repair the nurse call system, approximately two hundred stations; the tele-intercom system, approximately four hundred stations; and the paging system. We handle the computer repair and some programming; designing, building, and modifying of medical instrumentation to fit the needs of the medical staff; and the evaluation of new equipment. And we provide electrical safety education when requested."

Because Children's is a specialty hospital and research-oriented, "we have as much equipment here roughly for a 210-bed hospital as you probably find in a five hundred-bed general hospital." As an example, Wispolis explains that gravity is normally all that is necessary in providing medication or fluids IV to an adult patient, but because precise measurement is so much more important with children, infusion pumps—devices used for the introduction of medication into a human being—are almost always required. Children's has 275 infusion pumps in operation (some patients require three and four different medications simultaneously) at any given moment. Infusion pumps also provide the capability of electronic surveillance: an alarm goes off when the fluid runs dry.

The Biomedical Division also maintains all the physiological monitoring equipment, such as the electrocardiograph, as well as electrosurgical equipment for the cutting of tissue, such as the cauterizing needle employed so skillfully by Marc Rowe upon Danielle Burdette. Working with the Chairman of the Department of Anesthesiology, Wispolis has helped to design and build a Neuromuscular Evoke/Response system to aid anesthesiologists in determining the patient's depth of sedation.

Design and maintenance of operating room and diagnostic equipment is an essential part of the job—even if it means going right where the action is and even when that action is taking place directly in the operating arena. Once, about a year before the completion of the Main Tower, Domenic Costa, thirty-eight, manager of Engineering Services, employed at Children's for eighteen years, received a STAT (emergency) call on his pager—he receives twenty-five to fifty pages a day—to the OR. The circulating nurse was waiting for Costa when he arrived, lugging a toolbox. Immediately, he was outfitted with scrubs, mask, hat, and footcovers and escorted inside, in the middle of a tense and dangerous open-heart procedure.

The patient was on a water bed, Costa recalls, requiring cold water to slow circulation in order for the doctors to repair the heart. Warm water was then supposed to be employed to return circulation to normal, but the hot water supply line had clogged. Costa, who had often tinkered with the aging plumbing in the old building, immediately recognized the problem. Over a period of years, lime in the water can cause the copper bellows in the mixing valve to jam, he explained, "so I began beating on the pipe with a wrench. The surgeons thought I had gone crazy, but I knew what I was doing. In a little while, the bellows opened and the hot water began to flow.

"But then the surgeons wouldn't let me leave, just in case it happened again." As the surgery continued, Costa used the OR phone to call for backup assistance. "We got a garden hose, rigged it up to the scrub sink. If the line had clogged again, over the next hour and a half that the operation went on, we would have been ready."

Costa and his men were also ready just a couple of years ago, when the city reservoir a few miles north of the hospital, which supplies water to the entire facility, was inadvertently shut down, at 3:30 A.M. Costa knew that there was water in the immediate vicinity of the hospital for emergency purposes, and he also knew that people in the community would help a hospital in distress— especially Children's Hospital. He drove to the local fire station, woke up the men on duty, explained the situation, and requested as many fire hoses as they could spare. He then directed his men, who had been roused out of bed, to string the fire hoses up and down the stairwells, connecting every floor in the building to the hospital fire pump.

While Costa was jerryrigging his temporary water system, more of his men, who had volunteered for work, began packing large bottles of distilled water on their backs for delivery to the OR and hauling steel drums filled with water around the building for flushing the toilets. "We fed the building with water, and all with little inconvenience to normal routine," says Costa, "for three days and nights, until water service was restored."

Although Children's is totally reliant on the city of Pittsburgh for water, the institution is equipped with a backup generator for electricity, which will automatically go on-line the moment the local public utility experiences any problem posing a threat to the hospital's electrical supply. The emergency generator, powered by diesel fuel stored in a 4,000-gallon underground tank, will operate "indefinitely," according to Stranahan. "We recently cranked them up in a test that went on for ninety-six hours."

There is also a 5,500-gallon central system for the supply of liquefied oxygen, shared by Children's, Presbyterian-University, and Eye and Ear hospitals. Not only does this central system have its own backup, but Children's maintains a private supply just in case the system and its backup both falter. Other essential medical gasses include nitrous oxide, used to anesthetize patients, and nitrogen, which powers drills, saws, and most other surgical equipment in the operating room.

According to Stranahan, Facilities Management and Engineering Services touches and influences the life of every employee in the building, almost on a daily basis. "The fact of the matter is that somewhere along the line you will call me for something, whether it's to change your light bulb, fix your door, hang a picture on the wall, or stop the water suddenly leaking from the ceiling. Inevitably, you will call us, and before you know it, we'll be there."

Chapter 28

PREPARATIONS for Christmas at Children's Hospital start early—right after Thanksgiving—just as they do in most suburban malls and shopping districts. In addition to the activities centered on the Free Care Fund, with the Pittsburgh Press Old Newsboys' and radio campaigns, and the KDKA-TV telethon, the season comes alive in the hospital cafeteria with a Christmas castle of canes, candies, and crackers—a joint effort of patients on five hospital units. The cafeteria offers an array of colorful holiday cookies for sale, while children representing different schools and religious congregations begin to decorate the cafeteria windows in competition for a prize in a contest that ends December 15. There is also a holiday door-decorating contest for the staff of the hospital—an honor captured in 1988 by the secretaries in Marc Rowe's Department of Surgical Services.

On December 20, there is an employee holiday party, and the following day a hospital sleigh ride, but there is no more important sign of the arrival of Christmas than the rows upon rows of boxes wedged into every corner and crevice of Santa's Workshop or stacked along the corridors directly outside the workshop door. Here are toys, games, and gigantic stuffed animals donated not only by Pittsburgh-based organizations, but also by companies from throughout the United States that care about kids.

Santa's Workshop, which is actually a large conference room reserved for the Christmas season by the Child Life Department, "looks just like Children's Palace," according to Sue Baurle, who, as Santa's chief helper, may well have the best job in the hospital. Baurle unpacks the gifts purchased by the Child Life Department, for which she has worked the past seven years as an aide, and organizes them by age groups and categories.

The eight Child Life specialists who work with children throughout the hospital will then be able to come into the workshop and select five gifts for each patient—in response to a Christmas wish list each child has been invited to submit.

If there is one way to distinguish between a children's hospital and a regular health-care institution with a pediatric unit, it is the existence of an active and creative child life department, large and experienced enough to integrate the overall rhythm and beat of the hospital with the reality—both practical and frivolous—of the child's world outside. Although she is the only nonprofessional on the Child Life staff of nine specialists, most of whom have master's degrees in child development, Sue Baurle, currently attending night college for a bachelor's degree, is perhaps the most integral member of the team.

For Easter, Santa's Workshop will be transformed into the Easter Bunny's Den. A great deal of candy and toys is purchased and donated for the holiday season, but actually, Baurle says, toys are contributed to the hospital throughout the year by large corporations and private citizens alike, much of which cannot ever be used, however. "People clean out their garages and cellars and sometimes send things to us. We get tons of used stuffed animals," none of which can be given to the children because of the dangers of spreading infection and bacteria.

As Baurle sets up the Bunny's Den, the Child Life specialists carefully examine the patient's diet restrictions so that their Easter baskets will not contain candy and other foodstuffs that will be harmful to them. The Easter Bunny (actually Baurle in deep disguise) distributes the baskets to all patients on Easter morning. The hospital also has a great many costumes for kids to wear during Halloween, when all the patients, including those who are ventilator dependent, will canvass the hospital, trick-or-treating. Once again, the Child Life specialist protects the child by coordinating with nurses and other staff members so that each child will be given candies and other goodies in concert with dietary restrictions. Special events are routinely planned at Children's Hospital for all major holidays—Valentine's Day, St. Patrick's Day—whatever.

In addition to these events, one of Sue Baurle's more routine responsibilities is to host entertainers and other personalities who want to come into the hospital and visit some of the children. "A representative of the Pittsburgh Pirate organization will phone once every two weeks to offer the Pirate Parrot [the team mascot] and a player. I take them bedside, and they sign autographs. The Steelers will come once a year, during Christmastime." Mascots of national retail organizations, such as the Zayre Bear, are also frequent visitors. "About five years ago, there was a little boy, and the first time he saw me, I was coming through the hospital with Chuck E. Cheese. The next time he saw me I was alone. He said, 'Look, Mom, there goes Chuck E.'s mother.' That's why some of the nurses, to this day, call me 'Mrs. Cheese.' "

Mickey Mouse, accompanied by Goofy and Donald Duck, appears twice a year to say hello and to pass out Mickey Mouse ears to all the children. Mr. Rogers, a former board member of Children's Hospital, will come to visit kids on special request. (As a young man, Rogers studied at the University of Pittsburgh and Children's Hospital under the famous Benjamin Spock, who practiced at Pitt and Children's in the early 1950s. Jonas Salk was at Children's and Pitt at the same time, developing the polio vaccine, for which he was subsequently awarded the Nobel Prize.) Baurle, the only person ever to serve as Child Life aide at Children's, has also hosted Olympic Gold Medal winner Mary Lou Retton, and, "believe it or not, Sophia Loren was here three or four years ago. But meeting the real characters from Disney World is just probably the biggest thrill I have ever seen on kids' faces," Baurle says.

As part of her regular routine, Baurle visits each playroom early in the morning to clean equipment and put all the toys in place, ready and waiting for the Child Life specialists to begin their daily program of activities. Baurle also restocks supply cupboards in each playroom from four supply rooms that she maintains throughout the hospital. The supply rooms have games, organized by age groups, and videotapes; there is at least one VCR on each floor, especially effective for bedbound kids who cannot come into the playroom—along with many tapes, including one made by the children of the hospital, supervised and edited by Child Life. Baurle also feeds and cares for the gerbils, the only animal approved by the Infectious Disease Department to interact with patients.

One supply room is used exclusively for arts and crafts materials and "all kinds of weird stuff. Bubbles for blowing, for example. It's soothing for kids who can't even sit up in bed to have bubbles blown for them. Bubbles are a big winner in the holding area for kids just going into surgery because most of them are sedated and the bubbles help them quietly drift off." Other items include "wiggly eyes, the little eyes that squiggle. Glue them onto a Styrofoam ball and you've got an animal's head. Sequins and glitter are very popular at Christmas for making ornaments." Cooking supplies can also be found in the stock rooms, especially chocolate chips, cake mixes, and decorations, because if a child anywhere in the hospital has a birthday, a Child Life specialist will organize a group of children to bake a cake or cupcakes in honor of the occasion. Baurle will also purchase and wrap a special gift for each birthday child.

Stephanie Stein, director of the Child Life Department, explains that a birthday cake would be expected by children from parents and families in most homes, so why not in a hospital that exists for the sake of kids? There are toaster ovens, microwaves, and assorted cooking and baking utensils available in the playroom. The idea is to maintain normalcy, while occasionally arranging special activities and surprises to boost an ailing child's sagging spirits. For a teenager who missed high school graduation, the Child Life staff recently borrowed a cap and gown and convinced the principal to come into the hospital to bestow the degree personally. "In the winter, most children like to play in the snow," says Stein. "If we can't convince the docs to permit them to go outside for a few minutes, then we might bring some snow into the hospital for them to play in."

According to Margo Kennedy, who has worked at Children's Hospital for six years, each of the Child Life specialists is assigned a playroom or area of responsibility on each patient unit. There are also adolescent Child Life specialists for teens—regardless of unit or location—and another specialist in the ICU, as well as in the OR holding area. Kennedy, who is assigned to Unit 9 South, where most of the high-risk, trauma, and transplant patients are located, divides her job description into three categories. "One is to provide emotional support for patients, given what they are going through, that they are hospitalized and sick." (Social workers provide the same sort of support for parents and other family members.) Child Life specialists are responsible for communicating notes and ideas in a patient's chart, as will nurses, doctors, and other consultants called in on a case.

Second, it is her responsibility to see that a child's growth and development are ongoing, despite illness. A normal child (there is a separate Child Development Unit at Children's for patients suffering from more serious aspects of "developmental delay"), admitted to the hospital at two years old, who remains for six months because of a variety of complications, might well leave the hospital, given Kennedy's help and attention, with the age-appropriate skills of a two-and-a-half-year-old.

For older children, Kennedy will act as emotional counselor, while serving as liaison between patients and teachers, who will come into the hospital regularly to tutor school-age patients. The object is to facilitate a smooth return to normal life. There is even a Teen Lounge, supervised by adolescent specialist Lynn Mulroy, who is also active in the summer in Camp Can-Do, a two-week backwoods experience in eastern Pennsylvania for children recovering or suffering from cancer.

"Play is a child's work," says Kennedy, echoing Piaget, "and the place where they do their work is the playroom. The playroom is the child's emotional sanctuary at a children's hospital, a place where kids can feel safe." This leads to Kennedy's third and most vital role: child advocate, the protective screen and/or filter between the patient and the medical staff, primarily the doctor. Because she works so closely with children, Kennedy has come to understand their fears and inhibitions more than most adults and, as advocate, can help children more clearly communicate their needs and expectations. "I can be the words and the voice that states those needs for a four-year-old who doesn't have the verbal skills to do that for himself." She can also protect them from the persistence of physicians preoccupied with the patient's physical health who ignore emotional stability.

"Being a child advocate, one of the things I argue for on an ongoing basis for children is privacy. It is a long-standing rule in the playroom that medical procedures or exams are not allowed, no matter how harmless. She remembers a resident who walked into the playroom and was in the process of standing an eleven-year-old boy up against a wall in order to take photographs for cranial facial surgery. "It looked like the doctor was a cop, lining up a convict for a mug shot, and there were three other kids in the room, and they were all watching the process with great curiosity. At that point, the most important job I had was to advocate on behalf of the child to move the procedure to a private area. That kid doesn't have to feel like a freak—some animal in a zoo."

Medical discussions between anyone—doctor, nurse, parent, and child alike—are also prohibited in the playroom because children can be easily misled. Conversations about the health or future therapy for one child can be overheard and misconstrued by another child; imaginations will often run wild. Depending on their most recent experience, the sight of a nurse with an IV tray or a doctor in a white coat, with or without a needle, may be frightening. Pain and discomfort are hospital realities, but not in a playroom. "Kids can't do their work with one hundred percent energy and creativity if they are distracted—or frightened."

Encouraging a doctor or a parent to leave the playroom in order to discuss any aspect of the child's state of health is extremely difficult for the Child Life specialist. "Parents are anxious for information and don't want to be interrupted." Doctors are busy and they, too, have only one task in mind: to talk to the mother and/or father, answer the necessary questions, and continue dealing with the countless other items on their agenda. She will never forget the most intimidating confrontation she has ever experienced over the issue of the playroom as the child's emotional sanctuary. It was with Thomas Starzl, whose impatience is legend throughout the Pittsburgh medical center.

Starzl had walked into the playroom to examine the surgical dressing on a twelve-year-old girl. He was just starting to lift up the girl's pajamas when Kennedy asked him to take his work elsewhere. "I was terrified," she says. But he stopped what he was doing momentarily and stared up at Kennedy with a look of both impatience and curiosity, as if he really wanted to know why this was such an issue. "I explained that sometimes teenage girls might not like somebody looking under their pajamas in front of other kids in a very open place. Kids might feel private about their bodies. He turned to the patient and said, 'Is it OK with you if I look under your pajamas here in the playroom?' And she, of course, said 'Yes.'" What else could she say to the man who had saved her life?

"Then I was really caught," said Kennedy, "but then another idea came to me. I said, 'Well, sometimes there might be other kids, unlike this young lady, who might feel that way, and there also might be children in the playroom who might feel embarrassed or frightened by what they see." As Starzl stood and stared at her, Kennedy discussed for a few seconds longer the modesty and limited experiences of children and the stress under which they exist in a hospital setting. But at that point, Starzl had seen enough and was satisfied that the girl's wound was healing. He left the playroom and visited his other patients on the unit. Some minutes later, as he rushed toward the stairs, he passed Kennedy, who was standing in the corridor in front of the playroom, relating the confrontation to her partner. Suddenly, Starzl stopped and whirled around. "Oh-oh," Kennedy said. "Here comes trouble." But Starzl smiled. "Thank you for telling me that," he said.

Chapter 29

JUST as emergency rooms in adult hospitals are often ill-equipped to handle children properly, so too are many of the average transport systems that speed these patients to the ER door. According to Richard Orr, the intensivist who directs the Children's Hospital transport team, one of the largest of approximately twenty-five pediatric transport teams nationwide, the average flight nurse may have been indoctrinated with only four or five one-hour lectures focusing on the care and treatment of children in distress, and the licensed paramedic, through a 1,600-hour training regimen, will have had a day, perhaps two, actually on the job with kids. Orr says that 10 percent of all hospital transports via ambulance were with children under four, and yet, according to a recent study in Los Angeles, 75 percent of all ambulances are not equipped with the specialized airway equipment required to help a child breathe.

Orr and ICU fellows Robert Dimand and Carol Singleton recently presented a paper reporting the results of the 507 nontrauma patients transported between July 1986 and June 1987. Although the amount of transports nearly doubled during the same period in 1988–89, the results are similar. Fifty-three percent of all transports were by helicopter, 6 percent by airplane, and 41 percent by ambulance, with an average response time (actually leaving the hospital after the call) of approximately 29 minutes by air and 33 minutes for ground transport. According to Dimand, the response rate could and should be better, but Children's transport is sometimes "bumped" by the higher-priority pediatric and adult trauma teams that share certain communications facilities and equipment in Pittsburgh.

Dimand feels that the efficiency of the transport team along with the image of Children's Hospital would be enhanced if the hospital owned its own helicopter. Helicopter transport is extraordinarily expensive—$2,600 per hour, not including the $400-per-hour charge for the transport team—but it has been repeatedly proved, says Dimand, that saving time can mean saving lives.

As beneficial as helicopter transport can be, nurses and doctors do not particularly relish the experience. Noise and vibration, along with the very close quarters, will frequently cause air sickness. "Everything jiggles," says head nurse Valerie Karr. "If you don't have everything tied down, you see it moving. If you put your pen on top of something, it's on the floor before you know it. If it's hot outside, it's much hotter inside. In the wintertime, even with the heat at full blast, your feet are cold as ice. The wind makes it much worse."

She remembers one helicopter transport during high wind. They arrived at the hospital where the pickup was to be made, stabilized the child, and took off. "We had used so much fuel fighting the wind that halfway there we had to stop and refuel. So then we had to unload the baby, because you can't fuel with a patient on board. On the way back, the doctor got sick, then I started getting sick. Then the patient got sick. Most people can pull themselves together, but when the patient gets sick in small quarters, and you can smell the vomit, compounded by wind and vibration . . . You just hold on tight, wait to see Pittsburgh in the distance, and hope you get home."

As of December 1988, the pediatric transport team had transported nearly 2,700 patients. Orr says that in most cases the transport team will accept patients only from other hospitals, occasionally at doctors' offices, or even at a child's home in exceptional circumstances. Because of the "golden hour" concept for trauma, accident victims usually cannot wait for the transport team to arrive on the scene.

When summoned, the Children's Hospital transport team, which consists of eight full-time nurses in full complement (one nurse and one doctor per transport), each with a minimum of three years' experience in the pediatric ICU, will travel with its own equipment—an isolette (which weighs 250 pounds), a portable ventilator, and whatever supplies are needed. The supplies carried by the transport nurse, in a 37-pound bag, according to Valerie Karr, include: two Ambu (breathing) bags; a variety of sizes of face masks, syringes, needles; Band-Aids; "reagent" sticks (to check glucose); IV bags; medications; suction equipment; restraints for tying down combative patients; gloves; blood pressure cuffs for every size of infant, child, and adult; a special laryngoscope (to examine the larnyx) with extra batteries; and pulse oximeters, which measure oxygen saturation. Aircraft and ambulances are equipped with suction machines, oxygen tanks, even refrigerators.

Although doctors, nurses, and respiratory therapists are the most visible members of the transport team, the vital link between the team and the hospitals that contact it are the dispatchers in the new $500,000 high-tech communications system room, equipped with a "conferencing bridge" allowing as many as twenty-eight doctors at Children's and at the referring hospital to communicate simultaneously. The communications system was actually designed by trauma team surgeons to make it possible for all potential specialists at Children's to consult with the paramedics on the scene or en route to the hospital. The dispatcher, laboring for hours in a tiny, windowless Communication Center jammed with equipment, monitors all conference calls, contacting and "plugging-in" other consultants as needed and subsequently arranging for the appropriate transport. For educational purposes, all such conversations, whether for trauma or transport, are automatically tape-recorded and simultaneously documented with notes compiled by the dispatcher on his or her personal log sheet.

Because of the critical nature of their role, providing information to and from all parties involved in either transport or trauma situations, each dispatcher at Children's has become a licensed EMT (emergency medical technician). "If necessary," says Darlene Opalko, director of the Communications Department, "we can deliver babies, intubate, or splint; we can do anything an EMT does, except ride in ambulances." Working on a rotating basis, the dispatchers will also operate the hospital telephone system; handle STAT calls, emergency "codes," and doctor pages; dispense and repair hospital beepers; and operate the Information desk at the front entrance.

A pediatrician accompanies the nurse on each and every transport. Second-year residents, who have completed neonatal training, are assigned duty for all newborns and infants under six months of age, while an intensivist—one of the fellows from the pediatric ICU—will be responsible for all transports for older children, who are much more likely to have more complicated problems. When a ventilator is needed, a respiratory therapist will also accompany the transport. The Children's Hospital transport team averages two transports a day—airplane, ambulance, or helicopter—and although 95 percent of the transports are within a hundred miles of the hospital, the team has traveled as far as the West Coast for patients in need of the special therapy Children's Hospital offers.

For the first transport, on December 23, a quick run to Forbes Regional Hospital, in Monroeville, Pennsylvania, not far from Pittsburgh, the ambulance driver momentarily lost his sense of direction and inexplicably drove an extra mile down the road. Siren blaring, tires screeching, we backtracked and pulled up at the ER entrance less than a half hour after leaving Children's. Despite the confusion, it was a fast run, says Arcangela Lattari, the second-year resident in charge, who calls herself Arc. "Too fast for me. Every time I do transport, I end up seasick."

"Which wouldn't be half bad if we lived in Florida," says transport nurse Bonnie Hogue.

"Don't tempt me," says Lattari. "I'll leave tonight."

The paramedics have jumped out of the ambulance, opened the rear door, and unloaded the equipment. The hospital security guard, expecting us, leads the way.

Rolling a portable isolette on a cart and carrying suitcases of supplies and equipment, we rush down the hall and into a tiny four-bed nursery. "You do enough of this," Lattari says, "makes you never want to have any kids."

The child we have come to retrieve was born two months prematurely and was in some respiratory distress. He is being transferred to the Children's NICU for observation.

A nurse tells Lattari, "Their mom and dad, they're a little bit different from most people. Even though the dad's a doctor, I think he's afraid of the kid, but they're real nice anyway. I think they are in shock. The pregnancy supposedly was going so smoothly. Then suddenly . . ."

Quickly, Hogue and Lattari transfer the infant to the portable isolette, but before leaving, we visit the mother's room, so that both parents can say goodbye. As we enter, the mother is on the phone, smoking a cigarette, wiping her red eyes with a wrinkled and balled-up handkerchief. Perhaps we have caught her at an awkward moment, for she seems embarrassed, backing away from the isolette. Hogue has opened a little door in the unit so that the mom can reach in to touch her tiny baby.

"He looks okay to me," says the mother, unwilling to move any closer.

The father is sitting at a table in the corner of the room, surrounded by dirty dinner dishes and a mound of wrinkled clothes. Despite the mess, the room is well appointed, with more of a resemblance to a hotel suite than a hospital area. "I'll be down to take care of things in the morning," he says. "First thing."

On the way back to Pittsburgh, it begins to snow. Lattari and Hogue watch the child in the isolette, while carefully ministering medication, talking quietly, periodically complaining about the swaying and bumping. The ambulance squeaks and shakes as we move rapidly down the road. The little baby remains undisturbed, periodically raising his foot and curling his tiny toes in a knot.

On the portable walkie-talkie, which all transport nurses carry, Hogue receives a call from the dispatcher at Children's Hospital, informing her of a transport pending in Tyrone, Pennsylvania, a tiny town near Pennsylvania State University, perhaps 125 miles east of Pittsburgh. "Tyrone must mean Rachel," says Hogue. "Little Rachel. She's got heart and lung problems. Lived for fourteen months in the RCU before her parents took her home. They live on a farm.

"The last time we got Rachel, we bypassed the hospital and landed in their hayfield. Her brothers and sisters went crazy; even Rachel thought it was fun." Hogue says that in the past two years in transport, she has landed in football fields and parking lots. "You never know where you might have to put down." At this point, it is not clear whether we will go to Tyrone by helicopter or airplane. She motions out the window at the gusty wind and snow. "Chopper pilots won't fly in weather like this."

The transport to Tyrone is still pending as we arrive at Children's, but we are immediately dispatched to the exact opposite end of the city for a child, also prematurely born, who turned blue and stopped breathing in a pediatrician's office. A local ambulance service was summoned to transport the child to the North Hills

Passavant Hospital ER to rendezvous with the Children's transport team.

We arrive at North Hills Passavant five minutes before the baby in distress. Business is slow in the ER during this evening so close to the holiday. Two respiratory therapists and four nurses are waiting in a semicircle around a newly made-up bed, like waiters and chefs at a fancy dinner. This is an unusual and intimidating show of force, says Lattari, nervous because they will all be watching her. There are Christmas decorations hanging from turquoise tile walls, illuminated with artificial light. The baby arrives, carried by the doctor.

Lattari immediately intubates the baby to assure safe and steady breathing. The intubation goes smoothly, but the procedure is always challenging in an infant because the trachea is so narrow— perhaps only an eighth of an inch. A danger in children is allowing the tube to go straight down, thereby hitting the second opening, which is the esophagus. But infants are usually easier to intubate than older children because, according to Robert Dimand, "they're not as strong and they don't have teeth." Dimand says that trauma teams, on the scene and pressed for time, often force, or "brutalize," the endotracheal tube in. You ask a trauma team member what kind of medication they used to intubate, "they'll tell you, 'Brutane.' But you better get the tube in. A paralyzed child cannot breathe without intubation."

After the intubation, as the respiratory therapist begins to administer oxygen, Lattari telephones Bill Simmons, the intensivist on call that night in the Intensive Care Unit, for instructions. Simmons suspects that the child's problem is RSV, a respiratory virus that particularly affects newborns in the cold months of winter (a hypothesis that subsequently proved to be accurate). He approves of the intubation and recommends that Lattari put in an intravenous line to stabilize the child even further before moving her back to the Children's ICU.

Putting in an A line, or arterial line, proves not to be nearly as easy as intubation. Back and forth, Lattari focuses attention on the child's tiny arm and leg, tapping the wrist and foot with a stiff forefinger, searching for a likely access vein. Utilizing needle after needle, Lattari attempts—unsuccessfully—to sink the line. Periodically, Hogue will lean over and wipe the perspiration-soaked hair from Lattari's eyes. Lattari has long and dramatic straight black hair, which seems to grow increasingly wild, shooting out in all directions, as she labors. Wrappers and plastic tops from fresh needles litter the bed. The baby is constantly kicking and crying, getting cold, losing body heat. The nurses look for a heat lamp. Lattari wraps a rubber tourniquet around the baby's forehead, searching for access in the larger veins in her tiny fuzzy scalp. Eventually, without success, Lattari asks the nurses to send for one of the anesthesiologists on call in the OR within the hospital. "Maybe he can help."

"Sometimes you will find that with your eyes closed, you could hit any single, chosen vessel with a needle at twenty paces," ICU fellow Denise Goodman later explains to me. "Arterial line, venous line, putting a line in the umbilical vessels. Other days, you can try till you are blue in the face, and you just ain't going to hit it. You are cold."

The anesthesiologist arrives and quickly locates the access in the scalp for which Lattari had been searching. It takes him less than thirty seconds. He surprises himself.

"I never did an IV that small," says the anesthesiologist. "I hope it stays."

"It's okay," says Lattari. "Thanks very much."

A nurse comes in. "Can we tell the mother something? She's petrified out there."

"Tell Mom we were having trouble putting the IV in, but it's okay. It'll be all right. I'll come out and see her before we go."

In the waiting room, the mother, Kathy Cooksey, a twenty-seven-year-old elementary school teacher, explains: "The night before, Michele had had a couple of spells where she didn't breathe, and I called the pediatrician, who told me that newborns tend to stop breathing for very short periods. The next day, she had two more of those spells, and then at about four in the afternoon, there was a real bad spell. I got scared. I shook her. I squeezed her chest. I was yelling, 'Please breathe again, please . . .'

"I called the pediatrician again, and she said to come in. She couldn't find anything wrong, but we decided to send her to Children's for observation anyway. We called an ambulance, got her loaded up, and right before we were ready to take off, the ambulance attendant said, 'Wait just a minute; I want to go ask the doctor something.' Immediately, the doctor came rushing out because, in fact, Michele had had another blue spell, a serious one, and the attendant didn't want to alarm me. That's when we arranged to meet you people at Passavant."

As soon as the anesthesiologist disappears, the line he has inserted pops out. The nurses summon him again, but by the time he returns, Lattari has found a cooperative vein in Michele's wrist and quickly sinks the line. She phones Bill Simmons for instructions before leaving. The mother has asked to ride along in the front seat of the ambulance. The father, who is at home caring for the other children, will follow later in the family car.

As we speed along the roadway, sirens blaring, red ball whirling in the darkness, I ask the mom where she got her southern accent.

"Birmingham, Alabama."

"How long ago?"

"Seven weeks."

"Seven weeks?"

"Yeah," she says, glancing back at her newborn child with glazed and worried eyes. "Welcome to Pittsburgh."

At 10:00 P.M., we take off in an airplane to retrieve Rachel Houck, who is waiting at the Tyrone Memorial Hospital.

Flying in the plane is extremely relaxing. You can sit back and rest and think in the dark—listening, smiling, and nodding without having to respond if you don't want to, for the conversation is muffled by the roar of the twin engines. Before becoming involved in the medical world, I never gave much thought to the critical nature of a transport system. Not only have three children been helped within an eight-hour period, but simultaneously, in other parts of the country, more lives are being saved by the "golden hour" concept in trauma—rushing critical patients to qualified physicians and nurses before primary life-support systems begin to shut down. Working long and often lonely and boring stretches, transport nurses, trauma physicians, and procurement coordinators burn out quickly. These are heroes of high-tech medicine, men and women whose vital contributions are, unfortunately, frequently unrecognized or misunderstood.

Rachel, eight years old, has blue fingernails, a telltale sign of circulatory problems, caused by a weakened heart. She is coughing and hoarse, her lungs are filled with mucus, and she can't breathe without the help of a ventilator. She received a tracheostomy (insertion of a permanent artificial airway into the windpipe) when she was an infant. Although she attempted—unsuccessfully—to start school full-time this fall, she has been closeted at home for most of her life.

"Rachel's school experience actually didn't work out too well," says her mother. "I think she adjusted all right socially, but there were too many germs; she's susceptible to so many different infections." Mrs. Houck moves closer to the child to comfort her, as Bill Simmons begins to put in an intravenous line. Simmons taps the backs of Rachel's pale and fragile wrists, looking for access veins the same way Lattari did with Michele Cooksey.

Immediately, Rachel begins to cry. Her mother is kind but firm. "You know this has to happen, Rachel; either here or at Children's. Might as well get it over with now."

"It's amazing that everything happens at night," Bill Simmons comments. He is thirty-two years old and has recently been promoted to an attending at Eye and Ear Hospital in Pittsburgh—a position he will assume in a few months. "All the sick kids get sicker when the sun goes down."

Simmons experiences only minor delays, and although the IV goes in smoothly, Rachel is now screaming—a kind of hoarse and soundless scream, muffled by the tracheostomy. Eventually, she settles down. She says to her mother, "I'll be ready in two days."

"What's in two days?" Simmons asks.

"I told Rachel I'd call him up, and tell him to drop off all her presents at Children's Hospital," says Mrs. Houck.

"Him?" asks Simmons, smiling as if he didn't really know the identity of Rachel's secret benefactor.

"Santa Claus," says Rachel. At the sound of his name, she tries to sit up and smile, but she slumps heavily, in a fit of coughing.

Rachel looks cozier and more comfortable as the sedative Simmons has given her for the flight back to Pittsburgh begins to take effect. As we load her bed into the ambulance to return to the airport to pick up our transport, Rachel once again begins crying. Slowly and helplessly, she reaches out to her mother, who must remain at home for another day to care for the other three children in the family. She will join Rachel on Christmas at Children's. Momentarily, their fingertips touch. Then with tears streaming down her cheeks, Kathy Houck turns her back and walks away.

Even at 10:30 P.M. on Christmas Eve, we're off on a transport, this time to Sewickley Valley Hospital, another suburban hospital, for a teenager, sixteen, who got drunk, fell, and slammed his head against a parked car. The transport nurse is Lisa Shapiro. Intensivist Josephine Fratilio, who has come to Children's Hospital from her home in Puerto Rico on a two-year fellowship, is the pediatrician in charge.

"Anybody want to sing Christmas songs?" says the ambulance driver, as we speed along the highway.

"Only if it's in Spanish," says Fratilio.

"We just returned from a drug overdose," says Shapiro, "so to tell you the truth, even though the kid was okay, I don't much feel like singing."

"Actually, it wasn't so bad," said Fratilio. "If it hadn't been so dangerous, it might have been kind of funny." The child was only nineteen months old. He had accidentally swallowed 140 milligrams of Ritalin by mistake—the normal adult dose is 30.

"The kid was fine," said Fratilio. "Just dancing and dancing."

"He bit my finger," says the ambulance driver.

The city is quiet and dark on this holiday night, and the roads are empty, so we're traveling fast. "We're cooking," says the driver. Periodically, he will roll down his window and yell at the cars as he forces them aside. When we go under the bridges, the siren echoes as it screams.

"This boy we are going to get must be in trouble if they called us out tonight," the ambulance driver says.

"Yeah, this is an adult hospital. They should be able to care for him there," says Shapiro.

"As I understand from the dispatcher's report," says Fratilio, "he fell against a parked car. Originally, as they brought him to the ER, he could remember everything, but slowly he began to blank. He's being 'bagged' [an ambu bag; somewhat of a portable, hand-operated ventilator] right at this moment."

The boy's name is Mike, and there's blood caked all over his face; he is in a corner room in the ER—the only one of seven such rooms occupied tonight. The mother stands at the foot of the bed holding onto her son's bare feet. She is chewing gum, staring at his face. She wipes an occasional tear from her eye with the back of her hand. The nurse tells her not to worry. "Your son will be all right."

Quickly and quietly, Shapiro and Fratilio begin to tie the boy down, but as expected, the moment he senses their presence he begins to squirm and fight. "Calm down, Mike. You're okay, Mike. Calm down. Everything is fine," Fratilio and Shapiro reassure him.

Now Mike is bagged. Fratilio is holding his forehead; Shapiro takes his blood pressure. The two women joke about Mike trying to pull out the tube, figuring that they will get him to stop by relaxing him, making him feel comfortable, as if he were with friends. But he is unimpressed and keeps on fighting.

"Mike, I'm just putting a blood pressure cuff on you. Mike, stop this. Everything is okay," says Shapiro.

For ten minutes, the battle of Fratilio and Shapiro versus Mike rages, but when both his mother and the paramedics join the tussle, Mike immediately gives in. He is tied on the bed and hoisted into the ambulance. The red ball flashes, the sirens blare, and again, the ambulance cuts through the night.

In a few minutes, Shapiro calls the base dispatcher at Children's to report an ETA, then quickly signs off.

"You didn't say 'Merry Christmas,' " says Fratilio.

"Oh yes," says Shapiro. "It's just about Christmas."

"It's actually twenty-three minutes past midnight."

"Oh well," says Shapiro. "I forgot."

Part VI

Going Home

SENIOR surgical resident Steve Teich will usually begin his day at Children's Hospital at 6:00 A.M., leading a group of seven junior surgical fellows and rotating residents through a whirlwind tour of the hospital to examine and plan the day's treatment for the patients—eighteen on this day—for whom the Department of Surgery is currently responsible. He enters the Neonatal Intensive Care Unit (NICU; Teich calls it "Nick-U") and says to the first resident he sees, Joe Collela, the young man who had assisted with Danielle Burdette's surgery, "Speak!"

The Department of Surgery, with Marc Rowe as its chief, is responsible for all surgical patients in the NICU—Rowe is the surgical director of the NICU—while Brad Fuhrman, a neonatologist, serves as medical director, responsible for all other patients in the unit. As one of his many accomplishments, Rowe is credited with establishing the NICU when he arrived at Children's in 1980.

As we walk around and look at the little "peanuts" nestled in tiny incubators, Collela or one of the other residents discusses treatment plans for the day, as well as any concerns that the parents have expressed about their child. The NICU dispensed with, the group rushes, en masse, with the tails of their white lab coats flapping, to the Respiratory Care Unit (RCU, or "Rick-U") to see Danielle Burdette.

Despite the threat of infection, Danielle is recovering nicely. Teich notes that the wound has healed smoothly, that the drainage tube has been removed. Unfortunately, Danielle has been subjected to one additional surgery three weeks after Rowe's procedure: the insertion of another stent—the fourth over the past year. Sooner or later each of the other stents had become ill-fitting and troublesome, just as her tracheostomy never seemed to work for very long. This is the lesson that parents are forced to learn about chronically ill children and high-technology surgery and treatment, the same lesson with which transplant recipients and their families are continually confronted: that the initial diagnosis is, more often than not, only the beginning of a long series of problems that will stem from complications of treatment—from medications or, as in this case, from therapeutic surgery. In characteristic straightforward form, Debbie Burdette had already begun dealing with one major complication of treatment, Danielle's inability to speak. Lying on the chair adjacent to Danielle's bed, where Debbie will often sleep, is an instructional book entitled *Learning to Sign.*

Teich examines Danielle quickly, carefully bending over her bed so as not to awaken her. His clothes are rumpled and wrinkled, his striped tie is looped loosely in an old-fashioned Windsor knot. Although he is balding and overweight, he has a pleasant and open smile, cheerfully honest. On his cluttered desk in the office in the Department of Surgery, which he shares with two other pediatric surgical residents, are two photographs—the only two photographs—and both photos are of little Danielle Burdette.

After Teich's examination of Danielle, we head up to the units, or "floors," beginning on 10—the infant floor—and start to work our way downward. The hospital in the morning is shadowed and eerie; the lights are turned low, and most of the rooms are dark. On Unit 9 South, as on the other units, the lights will be turned on after the nurses working the oncoming day shift take the report from those who are just completing night turn. To save time and trouble, the night charge nurse has interviewed all of her nurses on the floor, then dictated her findings into a tape recorder. Before assuming responsibility, the day-shift nurses quietly listen to the tape, noting vital information, patient by patient, as reported by the charge nurse. It is a rare period of relaxation before the frantic pace of the upcoming day.

A few minutes after the report is complete and the nurses take the floor, the mother of an eight-year-old named Joel, flown to Pittsburgh from Israel for an emergency liver transplant, greets veteran RN Cheryl Craig by motioning to the bathroom.

"Oh, you left me a present," says Craig, understanding the signal immediately. She retrieves a tray of excrement and walks out of the room and down the hall into the specimen room.

"This is my favorite part of the job," she says with a straight face, checking the stool carefully for blood. She has also taken a urine sample, which she holds up in the air, cocking her head, and examines with a wary eye. "Looks good."

Returning to Joel's room, Craig records vital signs onto the chart, commenting about the importance of family support in enhancing the transplant recipient's recovery, as well as a sense of religion. "A lot of people suddenly get religion when they come here," she says, "but long-term religious conviction has a lot to do with how these people survive."

Joel's mother, clad in black, an Orthodox Jew, agrees. "It's so empty the life, without belief. You believe in God, then God will help you. Religion is a happy life."

"He reads all day," says Craig, referring to Joel. "Doesn't he watch TV?"

"Not nice things on TV," the mother replies.

Joel, short and twiglike after years of suffering from cystic fibrosis, remains oblivious to the conversation, reading his prayerbook, with his yarmulke almost dwarfing his tiny head. Joel is only three days posttransplant, but because of the high cost of the Intensive Care Unit (as much as $5,000 a day, depending on treatment, medication, and the diagnostics required) and the frequently overcrowded conditions of the unit (sometimes there aren't enough beds or nurses to deal with the incoming flow of patients requiring critical care), everyone involved (nurses, doctors, families) have been attempting to move patients onto the floors as fast as possible. This requires great flexibility on the part of the 9 South nursing staff, the ability to assume the role of an ICU nurse instantly without support of the ICU doctors, while at the same time caring for patients from other services, such as Neurosurgery and Trauma.

Now Craig begins the process of dispensing medications. At this stage in his illness, Joel must take twelve different "meds" at night and another dosage of the same meds in the morning.

Craig begins looking for the keys to the medicine cart. To protect against careless loss or theft, only one set of keys exists, for which every nurse on the unit seems to be constantly and fruitlessly searching. After she tries a dozen different predictable "hiding places," she discovers the keys in the general vicinity of where they belong—on the counter at the nurses' station.

After dispensing medications to her patients, Craig calls the pharmacy to order some of the meds that must be refilled for the cart. She then phones "escort" to retrieve the medicine—the most important being cyclosporine for Joel—and deliver it to 9 South. In the course of her work, she has accidentally spilled some of this precious oily medication onto her hands.

"Someone around here is doing a study to see how much cyclo we can absorb in our skin," she tells me. She is not certain of the purpose of the study but speculates jokingly that because one side effect of cyclosporine is excessive hair growth, Sandoz, the manufacturer, might be searching for a cure for baldness. "If I grow hair on these hands," she remarks, showing her pink, flat palms, "I'll go down in history."

Now she crosses the corridor and urges her other two patients, both named Brian, to begin washing up for the day and changing their clothes. Brian Number One doesn't know if he has any clean clothes, so Craig opens his suitcase and discovers a whole wardrobe. She selects an appropriate outfit, then, as he goes into the bathroom, she strips his bed. While he is washing, she rushes down the hall, dumps his soiled sheets in a closet, retrieves a fresh set, and begins folding and tucking crisp sheets and pillowcases.

Craig has to help Brian Number Two to dress, because he is still weak from surgery. But first, his IV pole has to become free from where it is tangled between the bed and the cart holding the computer he and Brian Number One were using late last night.

"Did you brush your teeth?" she says to Brian Number One, who emerges from the bathroom rather quickly.

"No, I guess I didn't. I guess I have to go back and do that."

"Well," she says, "let Brian [meaning Brian Number Two] brush first."

"I will brush," says Brian Number Two, "but I hate this Crest."

"But this Crest is bubblegum-flavored," says Craig.

"I don't care," says Brian. "I want my own toothpaste from home."

Soon it is time to give meds to Brian and Brian. Once again, she searches for the keys to the medicine cart.

"Keys, keys," she says walking toward the nurses' station. She finds the keys, unlocks the medicine cart, collects the medications she requires, drops the keys on the front desk, then returns to the Brians' room.

A few minutes later, as Craig is helping Brian Number Two dress, another nurse walks into the room to offer her the keys. "Here you are."

"If I wanted the keys I would have asked," says Craig, impatiently.

"Well, I thought you did ask."

The nurse stomps out of the room, nearly smashing into Teich, who has, in less than a half hour, discussed with his residents each and every patient attached to their service. Now, gathered in the corridor near the nurses' station on 9 South, "as good as any place to meet," they begin to discuss the OR schedule—the scheduled procedures—and decide which residents will scrub with which surgeons on which cases.

What's interesting to note about both Cheryl Craig's and Steve Teich's first hour of work each morning is how fast they move and, especially with the surgeons, how fast they can talk—so fast that I have difficulty understanding everything they say. This is only the second day for this group of residents to be on-service, and so they have not yet learned to communicate efficiently with Teich and each other.

Teich has a quick exchange with a resident named Rosenberg. They're talking about a patient who's just come into the hospital with abdominal pains and respiratory distress and they can't quite figure out why. Rosenberg says, "Maybe she's having her period."

"She's eight years old," says Teich.

"Well, then," Rosenberg replies, "maybe not."

Twenty minutes later, Teich is in the OR, about to assist attending surgeon Don Nakayama with the insertion of a central line for hyperalimentation (intravenous nutrition) for a child who cannot digest his food. As Teich scrubs, he talks about the upcoming cases for the day and the possibility that he may be able to do a circumcision (the case has yet to be assigned). He jokes that as soon as he finishes his fellowship, in order to get into the lucrative circumcision market, he's going to have business cards printed, reading: "Every kid deserves to have surgery by age six."

Teich is suddenly paged to the ER to see a child in severe respiratory distress. The doctors need IV access—and they need it STAT (quickly). As we rush into the room, the child, who is very small, is covered with blood. His skin is blue. Teich comments calmly to no one in particular that it is very difficult to get a "line into a kid who is so dehydrated," but he subsequently sinks the line in a matter of a minute with a couple of quick cuts from a glittering scalpel.

Teich is paged to the holding area, where a ten-year-old girl with an emergency appy has been transferred from the ER after having been transported to Children's from another hospital.

Suddenly there are three simultaneous conversations going on. Teich is talking to the patient and asking her questions. The anesthesiologist is talking to the parents, explaining what will happen to their child and why they must sign a consent form. The two nurses—the one who accompanied the child from the ER and the one who accepted her into the holding area—are also talking.

Teich turns away from the child and begins addressing the nurses. He must know how much the patient weighs ("thirty-three kilos," they tell him) in order to know how much antibiotic should be prescribed. The correct dosage is computed by Teich on the pants of his scrubs with his marker.

The fact that the ten-year-old was not given antibiotics immediately upon being admitted for surgery has made Teich very unhappy, for this was the responsibility of the surgical resident who had initially examined the child in the ER before admitting her. Teich complains that it seems as if half of his day is eaten up safeguarding patients against residents' mistakes. "These doctors are experienced but not in pediatrics."

Teich returns to the OR in time to see the child who had been about to get the central line now being rolled into the recovery room; Nakayama has completed the job. A new patient is now being rolled into OR #7 for an anoplasty (plastic surgery of the anus), required to permit the child to control his bowels more easily. This is an unusually complicated procedure because a great deal of scar tissue exists from a previous surgery and Nakajama has never performed it exactly this way before. Rowe has written a number of articles about the procedure, and so Rowe and Nakajama have already conferred. Although Nakajama has invited Teich to assist, he is expecting Rowe to take a quick look before starting.

Nakayama has arranged the child on his stomach, his anus tilted upward on slabs of sponge rubber. Teich, meanwhile, has drawn a line with his marker to guide first cut. But when Rowe arrives, he's not in agreement. Rowe and Nakayama begin to talk about the entire procedure, while Teich backs off a polite distance, commenting, "I'll give them five minutes, and they'll be doing it together."

It actually requires only about thirty seconds to recognize that Rowe will be deeply involved in the procedure for the duration. Teich whispers out of the side of his mouth, "Very soon I'm going to make my gracious exit. I make it a practice," he adds, "not to involve myself when two attendings scrub."

Teich takes off his gown and slowly and quietly exits into the adjoining OR, where Sam Smith is removing the appendix from the ten-year-old girl.

"I thought you were in on it next door," says Smith.

"When two attendings scrub," Teich says, "there's no room for a resident."

Alice, the circulating nurse working that day with Nakajama and Rowe, comes into OR #7 to say, "Dr. Rowe wants you."

"Now what do they want?" Teich says.

"Did you get insulted and leave?" asks Rowe, as Teich returns.

"No," says Teich. "I thought you guys seemed to be having great fun."

Teich must go to the NICU to check the status of the little girl whose line went in for hyperalimentation. Despite the fact that he missed the surgery, the care and treatment of this patient is his responsibility. At the conclusion of the procedure, the ten-year-old appy will also be his responsibility, supervised by Smith, as will the little boy receiving an anoplasty by Nakajama and Rowe. In most hospitals, the residents, led by the senior resident of each service, follow through with the hour-by-hour and day-to-day care and treatment. The attending comes and goes as he or she chooses, rounding and consulting with residents, colleagues, other subspecialists, and parents, as needed.

Although this loose and unofficial system has been in place in teaching hospitals throughout the United States as far back as anyone can remember, it leads to a great many inexplicable and confusing delays and a multitude of discontented parents, who are often supplied with marginally different opinions and possible treatment plans from every resident, attending, nurse, and technician having contact with their child. As a teaching method, permitting interns and residents to practice with competent supervision and backup, the system seems to work well—but at a certain sacrifice for the patient and family. Transmitting infection from patient to patient is also more of a possibility in a large facility with patients from all spectrums of society and with many different anomalies and infections.

A community hospital, with only a few residents and a small teaching program, often managed like a hotel because of its "for-profit" orientation, will undoubtedly provide more efficient and perhaps more affable service, with food and accommodations frequently of superior quality. On the other hand, if complications occur, if special procedures are required, university-affiliated institutions are much more capable of response. Selecting a hospital for surgery is a decision taken too lightly by consumers, content to follow the advice of their doctors, who may not be as well informed as they ought to be about the treatment after surgery and the backup capabilities of the institutions (many doctors have privileges in three or four hospitals) in which they operate.

After discussing the treatment plan with the charge nurse and the nurse assigned to the care of the child in the NICU who received the central line for hyperalimentation, we go for our own hyperalimentation—coffee. Teich drinks coffee as if he is quenching his thirst on a hot summer day: three or four quick gulps and it's gone. "When I'm home," he says, "I never drink coffee. I think I do it here because it's something to do."

Teich says he never had much desire to be a doctor. "Ever since I was a little kid, I wanted to be an engineer—since I was five years old. In fact, I went through Rensselaer Polytechnic Institute, which is the oldest engineering school in the country. I actually have two engineering degrees—biomedical engineering and materials engineering. I eventually went into medicine because I had a roommate in college who was pre-med, and he got me interested. I got him interested in engineering, and he eventually went into chemistry.

"I went to medical school in Buffalo for four years, and I knew immediately I wanted to go into surgery. My mother used to say she couldn't understand how I could do surgery, because as a kid I used to faint at the sight of blood. In fact, at the beginning of my exposure to surgery, I couldn't sit and watch an operation because the blood made me sick. It took me about two weeks to get used to it, forcing myself to sit in surgery for ten-minute increments and work my way up to an hour, watching operations. Today I can watch somebody bleed to death.

"Blood doesn't bother me anymore," says Teich, "but I can't stand infected toenails, and I can't stand broken fingers. Even today those two things will make me sick right off the bat. In fact, the first time I worked in a doctor's office—in your third year in medical school they have you work with a doctor—I was asked to clip some toenails on a patient who was infected, and I fainted in the examination room."

Teich is not married, and he has no children, "But I'm in the market for both—or either." With college, medical school, surgical residency, and then his pediatric surgical fellowship at Children's, he has been in training for his entire adult life. Most of his contemporaries at Children's had fallen in love and gotten married in or directly after medical school. Suzanne Ildstad actually went through two pregnancies during her residency. Most doctors, men and women alike, want to begin families before assuming their first positions as attendings—a time when their work, both clinically and scientifically, will really begin to count in terms of income, advancement, and reputation.

According to Marc Rowe, however, a very alluring woman has already staked a claim on Steve Teich: Danielle Burdette. Rowe said that over the past few months since her surgery, Danielle has become completely enthralled with his chief resident. When Teich walks into the RCU, Danielle's eyes follow him from bed to bed; when they converse in a group, Danielle will only listen to what Teich has to say; her hand automatically reaches out to stroke his arm, or her head somehow finds a way to rest on his shoulder.

Later that same day, during a lunch break with Rowe, I described an interesting scene I had observed relating to little Joel on 9 South. Joel's father, a rabbi in Israel, in his traditional black hat and coat, with his long beard and sidelocks, had been waiting for an elevator. When the elevator door opened, he was suddenly confronted with the father of another transplant patient, with a long beard and sideburns, garbed from head to toe in unassuming black. This man, however, was Amish. The two fathers stood and stared at one another for an inordinately long time—perhaps thirty seconds—without moving, knowing that they were obviously not of the same religion but sensing that their unique ways of life and feelings about the Deity were amazingly compatible. For all the problems posed by high-tech medicine, technology in many ways has helped bring together children and adults with contrastingly different cultures from throughout the world. Children from Peru, Argentina, Saudi Arabia, Italy, Greece, and Ireland have received liver transplants at Children's Hospital and lain side by side in the ICU or in rooms on 9 South.

Tabatha Foster, Starzl and Rowe's longest living multivisceral transplant, had united the black community in Pittsburgh in a very special way, said Rowe, bringing together ordinary citizens with black members of the media and black athletes from the Steelers and the Pirates—many of whom pledged financial support. Because Rollandrea Dodge, the second multivisceral transplant recipient, had been a Navajo Indian in a city with a very small Native American population, the support had not been as strong, but over the past few weeks, Rowe had learned a great deal about Indian culture.

Rowe said that the first time he and Starzl had "reexplored" Rolly after the initial transplant surgery, he had returned to the waiting area to give a report to the parents, but they were nowhere to be found. Instead, he saw three elderly Indian women with very passive expressions on their dark and wrinkled faces. He began to explain what had happened, but clearly their minds were elsewhere. Finally he asked, "Where's the mother?"

One of the women looked up briefly and replied: "She's sweating." Rowe realized that she was referring to the religious custom of heating stones, making steam—as in a sauna bath—and praying. "At first I had been angry when they were not around at such a crucial time, but then I realized that they were doing in their very own way what they could do to make their daughter better."

On another occasion, soon after the transplant, Starzl and Rowe had wanted to reopen the wound for an exploration. Cindy, Rolly's mother, was in the room when he arrived, but after Rowe asked for permission to do the exploration, she pointed at a "very official-looking Indian with a briefcase" who had just walked in the door. "Explain to him what you want to do."

Rowe explained, as requested. The Indian listened carefully, and then replied, "I think I can help you."

"He opened his briefcase, and then started taking out feathers and bones and old relics and other instruments," said Rowe. "This was the tribe medicine man. He actually did a little dance and moved around on his feet, said a prayer, began a chant while I stood there and watched. That's how I got permission."

A couple of years earlier, Rowe had performed emergency surgery on an Amish child who had been "a real disaster case. I worked and slaved and somehow nursed the kid back to health and sent him home. But the parents, through the long ordeal, were very quiet and very straight-faced, unsmiling and unthanking. They were civil at all times but never friendly. As soon as the child was well, they left without a word—and that was that." A year later, the Amish family returned and approached him in the same straight-laced and unsmiling manner. "They stood there in front of me," said Rowe, "and quickly, without any pretense, presented me with this beautiful

Amish patchwork quilt that they had made in the year since their child had recovered. They turned around and walked away so fast I hardly had the chance to thank them."

After gulping his cup of coffee, Steve Teich hurriedly returns to the action in the OR. "I don't like missing anything going on," he says.

Here is a child with a duodenal web causing a bowel obstruction, thereby making digestion impossible. Teich has never seen such a web, although he has read about them, so he goes to get his camera. In his office, he picks up his mail. "I get about three letters about jobs every week these days." His fellowship ends in about five months. "That's one thing about this fellowship. You know you're going to get work afterward." A Brooklyn native, Teich's objective is to get a good job in the Northeast—Boston, Philadelphia, Connecticut, or New York. (As it turns out, he will eventually end up with placement in Columbus, Ohio, where Marc Rowe first trained.)

Back into the OR, Teich takes his photo, then remains to observe and instruct the resident, Dr. Rosenberg, who is assisting with the closing after the gastric web has been removed. Teich emphasizes the importance of tight careful stitches, neat, high up on the skin, not too deep.

Teich says, "The only thing the patient sees at the end of the operation is a scar. When people need a pediatric surgeon, a friend will say, 'You go to Dr. So-and-So because he did a great job on my son.' What they really mean is, he did a great job on my son's scar. That's what a parent sees. The scar. They don't know about anything else unless there are complications."

It is now 1:10 P.M. and Teich helps the nurse push the gastric web into Recovery. Teich or one of his residents must accompany all patients from the OR to Recovery and to the ICU or NICU, to be on hand just in case of trouble. The "intensivists" assume responsibility (actually, it then becomes a dual responsibility, since the patient will also be under the overall supervision of the surgical attending) once the transfer has been complete.

After monitoring the child's status for fifteen to twenty minutes, watching carefully for any possible complications, Teich heads for the ICU to look in on the child in the ER for whom he provided IV access earlier in the morning. "When I saw how blue he was, I really thought that this kid would die. I had to be especially calm, so as not to alarm anyone else."

The child will probably not die now, but evidently the parents are well aware of the critical nature of the situation, for they have requested a clergyman, who is now kneeling at the bedside, clasping the hands of the mother and father, softly reciting a prayer of gratitude.

Meanwhile, Sam Smith has completed his appy and has accompanied the patient to the ICU, conferred with the parents, then returned to the NICU to round on some of his other patients. He points to the stuffed animals at the foot of almost every child's bed. "Sometimes there are so many animals, you can't find the patient."

Now Marc Rowe arrives; he has left Nakayama alone to finish the anoplasty. There are dark umbrellas under his eyes and a dirty stubble of beard on his cheeks and chin. He says he left the house at midnight yesterday, the evening of his thirty-second anniversary, to return to care for Rollandrea Dodge. "She's been bad," he says. "The black wings have been hovering over her for a few days."

"I thought you were going out of town," a nurse comments.

"Some people work when they are not supposed to," Rowe replies.

Smith says, "We tried to persuade Dr. Rowe to wean himself from the hospital, a little at a time, so that he could have a few days with his family without feeling guilty. It's hard for him to break away. He gets totally involved with patients like Rolly.

"Dr. Rowe is the patron saint of the lost-cause patients. If you ever get over your head with a patient, you just call him, because that's what Dr. Rowe loves best. He will leave his home and sit with you and help you with the patient for as long as you need him. Longer. He just really gets into it. His hair stands up on end and he gets that wild-eyed Buckwheat look we all laugh about, and he's completely and utterly involved. He does this to the extreme, sometimes at the expense of the other patients that he happens to be dealing with in the hospital."

I accompany Smith to an examination room near his office to see an eleven-year-old boy with a splenic cyst that must be removed. His mother has brought him here from Franklin, about sixty miles north of Pittsburgh, for a second opinion concerning where and by whom the surgery should be done. One surgeon in Franklin has told the mother that he feels comfortable performing the surgery, while another recommended she have the procedure done at Children's. Neither are pediatric subspecialists. "I want to stay close to home, but I'm confused."

Smith discusses the development of this particular procedure.

"Up until fifteen years ago, people just took the spleen out. That was the safest thing to do. What pediatric surgeons discovered was that one out of every four hundred kids will be endangered with pneumococcus without the protection of a spleen. So now they try to retain the spleen if at all possible." Smith points out that he has done five of these operations in the past three and a half years and that children's hospitals "are experts in children." But then he waffles, "On the other hand, if you trust the guys up there . . ."

Obviously, Smith could have been more forceful and persuasive with the mother, "but I worry about pushing," he says. "If she had asked me what I would do, then I would have told her. Or if she had asked me to be honest or to cut the bullshit— But she didn't ask any of that. We doctors are accused so often of paternalism. I am very much aware of that label, and it makes me feel uncomfortable. I try as often as I can to step back and let the patient and family decide what's best for themselves. Remember, she didn't ask me. She clearly seemed to want to make the decision on her own."

At 3:00 in the NICU, rounding begins again. Teich is unhappy. He seats himself at the nurses' station but tells his assistant to proceed without him. "This rounding at 3:00 is ridiculous—none of the test results have come back. But it's something new that Rowe wants to try, because the residents have been complaining that they're unhappy with the service because they have to work so hard and stay so late each night.

"But there's a reason for it. You wait for the tests so that you can prescribe and plan future action with all of the information and evidence at your disposal. Anyway, last week, the attendings decided they were going to schedule afternoon rounds for three o'clock, because the residents were complaining and felt they were overworked. So this week we're into 'quality of life' in the surgical service. But I don't think it's going to last."

Teich says, "I'm watching, but I'm not participating. I can't tell Rowe, or any of the other attendings on the service, how wrong I believe this is, but I can sit back and not participate, and do my own rounds later on when all the tests are in, and make sure the patients are okay. Sooner or later the attendings will begin to see how wrong they've been about this early rounding. I call this 'my passive resistance.' "

At 3:20, Teich leaves the NICU to see a possible appy on 9 South, a fifteen-year-old with awful abdominal pains. As he examines the boy, the mother tells Teich in a whining, rapid-fire monologue everything she has ever learned about appendicitis, based upon her experience raising two children and reading magazine articles. Her scientific determination is that appendicitis is hereditary.

"But do you have any questions you want to *ask* me?" Teich asks politely.

"Will my son be home by the weekend?"

As we proceed down the hall after the examination, Teich comments that in his experience there are two telltale signs of trouble between doctors and the mothers and fathers of patients. "Whenever parents tell me rather than ask me about their child's medical problems, I'm in trouble. And whenever parents ask me before the diagnosis is confirmed and the surgery takes place if their kid will be recovered and home in their own bed by the weekend, I know that the trouble will be profound."

At 4:10, Teich begins rounding through the hospital with Don Nakayama, quickly updating Nakayama on the status of each patient. Nakayama is on call that evening. Teich will then round on his own, familiarizing himself with the work his residents have accomplished through the day and the possible problems and plans to be discussed at rounds the following morning. Teich will then go to his office, dictate letters, make phone calls, and deal with hospital minutiae before rounding a final time and finally returning to his tiny apartment three blocks from the hospital.

"I round so much every day," he tells me, "I get dizzy."

Chapter 31

I N the Respiratory Care Unit on the 6th Floor, Debbie and Danielle Burdette are trimming a Christmas tree. Danielle is growing rapidly, gaining height and weight, and Debbie must be getting stronger, too, for she is lifting her daughter up high so that Danielle can hang a glittering gold ball on the top branches. Debbie is stretching so high, in fact, that the hose connected to Danielle's tracheostomy periodically pops its connection to the ventilator, triggering a piercing and beeping alarm. Perhaps because she cannot speak, Danielle repeatedly brightens at the sound of the alarm, and from time to time she will mischievously attract attention by triggering the alarm button with her fingers when no one is watching.

Danielle knows very little about playing with other children her age, but she is a whiz at charming and captivating her adult audience, often teasing her entourage with misleading symptoms. Periodically, she will point insistently into her mouth until Debbie becomes concerned and begins searching for an obstruction in her throat. Or she will point down at her buttocks, a signal that she needs to go to the bathroom, and Debbie and a nurse will rush Danielle to the potty and pull down her dress. Minutes will pass and nothing will happen, until Debbie finally becomes annoyed—at which point Danielle will burst out laughing.

Meanwhile, a couple of floors below, in the tiny office the hospital has allotted to me for conducting interviews in private, Trish Cambron and I are waiting for Debbie Burdette to finish with Danielle so that our "farewell conversation," an event we had planned for a long time, could start. Trish had adopted a two-year-old Korean child, renamed Joshua, who had been dying in a rural orphanage, and brought him to Children's for lifesaving surgery. In the process, Trish, a strong-willed woman of thirty-eight who had become accustomed to getting her own way through most of her life, had clashed with another driven personality, Josh's surgeon, Marc Rowe. For most of the two years in which I "lived" at Children's in order to research and write this book, there was hardly a time when Trish Cambron and Marc Rowe were not either at odds with each other—or expecting to clash at any moment.

And yet they clearly admired each other for their equally impressive accomplishments, Cambron for her work with children and Rowe for his clinical and research achievements (he has recently been named the first recipient of the Benjamin R. Fisher Chair in Pediatric Surgery). They also shared a deep and unshakable respect for the superwoman of One Children's Place, Debbie Burdette.

It is important to point out that not everyone at Children's *liked* Debbie Burdette, for in her obsession to care for her child and literally to force Danielle to survive and mature, despite all obstacles and against all odds, Debbie had stepped on some toes, ruffled some egos. And because of her independence and her familiarity with hospital routine, Debbie was known to attract as friends other "rebellious" mothers, such as Trish Cambron.

It would not be fair to connect rebelliousness with righteousness arbitrarily, because some parents I observed, even those with justifiable questions and complaints, could be uncooperative and rude, exhibiting little empathy for the point of view of hospital personnel. What made Debbie so outstanding to so many people, in addition to the way in which she devoted herself to Danielle, was her uncanny ability to blend into the fabric of the hospital, to accomplish her objectives in a manner compatible with everyone else's personal and professional concerns. Her best and most unfailingly impressive quality was her understanding of the mechanics of passive resistance. Debbie Burdette hardly ever asked for favors, privileges, or even basic services. She simply waited for them, no matter how many hours or days the waiting required.

This may have been why Debbie was late for our farewell conversation—she may have been waiting for someone to fulfill a promise or complete a responsibility—or it might simply have been that, because of her years at Children's, she had no concept of any rhythm of life outside of "hospital time." She, like the doctors with whom she dealt, would arrive at her scheduled appointment when she got there.

This is not to say that Debbie had been made into an entirely new person at Children's, for in many respects she was as much the little girl today as when she had first arrived from St. Albans. Now, five years later, she only infrequently dared venture into the busy neighborhood around the hospital, essentially the University of Pittsburgh campus; nor was she the least bit familiar with the fashionable area around the Ronald McDonald House.

Every night, often very late at night, after Danielle was asleep, Debbie would join the other members of the secret subculture of mothers from Children's Hospital, gathered in the kitchen at Ronald McDonald House, and tell war stories about their day. They would joke and laugh and knit and smoke and scream and cry, and hope for better times in the coming months, when their children were well enough to return home. These sessions were cathartic and therapeutic, yet disturbing, sometimes lasting until 2:00 or 3:00 A.M.

Trish Cambron remembers once sharing a room with Debbie Burdette after one of these long late nights. Debbie was so nervous, so "jazzed up" by the heightened intensity of the hospital, that, upon arriving in the room, she switched on all the lights and cranked up the radio and the television before finally flopping into bed and closing her eyes. "If the room had been dark and quiet," Cambron commented, "Debbie would have been completely unable to sleep."

A couple of weeks before Christmas, the *Pittsburgh Press* had published a front page story focusing upon Danielle's long-term illness and Marc Rowe's ingenious surgical procedure to help her continue to grow and to breathe. Debbie approved of the photograph of a smiling Danielle, in a beautiful red Christmas dress trimmed with white lace, standing in a walker, under the impressive although misleading headline,

LOOKING HOMEWARD
Life-Saving Surgery Corrects Deformity

but she was not too happy about the questions the reporter had asked her. "I was trying to focus on the progress Danielle had made over the years, and all he wanted to write about was her handicaps, the things she couldn't do. I'm against that completely. It just seems to me that kids have enough trouble being on a ventilator without having people calling attention to it."

Debbie is referring to one of the supreme ironies of health care—the fact that although man can make all of this technological magic to save lives, he does not know what to do with the patient after the miracle has been achieved and the lives have been saved. This is a subject that has been weighing upon Debbie Burdette these past few months as she begins to plan to take Danielle home once again.

"I'm worried," Debbie announced, when she finally arrived at my office that afternoon, an hour and a half late. "Is Danielle going to get the opportunity to start school? There's no reason for her not going to school, unless people want to look at her as if she's dumb just because she's on a ventilator. There are people who won't give Danielle a chance to prove what she can do because she's handicapped."

According to Danielle's father, Danny, who commutes faithfully each weekend from St. Albans, when you see Danielle at home the last thing you notice is her handicaps, for she is a child who has learned to appreciate the more common aspects of life while understanding vividly the meaning of the word "fun."

Danielle's most prized possession at home is a very fancy four-poster bed. Last year, one of the merchants in town had read a newspaper story about Danielle, and decided to give her something really special for Christmas. Danielle had her choice of any toy she wanted, but somehow, unbeknown to Debbie and Danny, she had been leafing through a J. C. Penney catalogue and in the process had found an elaborate four-poster bed. That's what she wanted more than anything else in the world. The merchant was true to his word, and since being presented with the bed, Danielle does not permit anyone else to sleep or lie on it unless they arrange themselves at the foot of the bed. Throughout our conversation, Danny kept laughing and saying about Danielle, "She's bad. She's so bad," meaning that she was spoiled, that she gets away with murder with every member of the family, and that this was quite all right with him.

In contrast to his wife, Danny Burdette seems to be always smiling and easygoing, as if he has resigned himself to the fact that these are the cards that life has dealt him and sees no reason to complain. The only thing to do is to make the best out of a terrible situation.

Danny tells me he's in air-conditioning and heating, that he can get a job anywhere. But in the same breath, he says that with the expense of Danielle's continuous medical problems, they've lost everything they ever had. They had to take a $100 pay cut in order to qualify for Medicare payments, so instead of making $350 a week, he makes $250 a week. But it doesn't matter. "We've already lost everything, so what the hell." He smiles and shrugs.

You can tell that Danny has not fought the daily battle for his daughter's survival, for his face is wrinkle-free and he looks much younger than his wife, who is actually a year younger than he. He has escaped the weight of the constant and ever-demanding intensity of the experience. Danny has labored in a support position, while Debbie has engaged in regular combat on the front lines of Danielle's battle for life.

From the first moment I met Danny, he couldn't stop talking about how much fun Danielle had been for them the last time they took her home. They try to take her everywhere she wants to go at home—even horseback riding. Her grandfather has a little pony, and Danielle will ride the pony while Danny or someone else follows along holding all the equipment—the ventilator and the Power Pak—as she clops around the track in a circle. She went to a carnival once, and they put her on the merry-go-round, and she loved it so much she wouldn't get off. Even when the portable ventilator got stuck under one of the horses—"Horse nearly crushed the damn thing!"—Danielle just wanted to keep riding.

I asked whether people didn't look at them strangely sometimes, or whether Danielle didn't attract a great deal of attention with all the equipment hooked up to her, and he said that there were various reactions. Some people showed real concern about Danielle, and others backed off, giving them as much distance as possible. He remembers being in a shopping mall and overhearing a woman passerby say about Danielle, "What a pitiful creature."

Debbie turned on the woman; she was furious and her face was in a rage and she said, "No, Danielle is not pitiful at all. She's my daughter."

"And she isn't at all pitiful," Danny added. "She's just different. That's the only thing wrong with her. She's different from everybody else."

Debbie is at the threshold of the pursuit of her newest obsession: Danielle's education. She will not for a minute relinquish her dream to send Danielle to a "real regular" school "because I think she's entitled. A handicapped child is entitled to school just as much as a normal child. That's why a lot of these kids stay handicapped—and stay dumb. I don't think that they're dumb in the sense of being retarded. But they don't get the help that they need to make it through this world. The fact of the matter is you can't make it through this world if you don't have an education. And you can't put a tutor in the house, and say, 'Okay, this is your school. Now learn!'

"A tutor in the house is not school. A classroom with a bunch of slow and other handicapped kids is not school either. I want Danielle to go to a normal school, and I want her to lead a normal life. Her only problem is her speech; right now she can't talk. So I'm going to teach her sign language so that she is ready to communicate."

Debbie Burdette's steadfast and unwavering persistence is without doubt the primary reason that her daughter is alive today, and also without doubt the primary reason that the people at Children's Hospital have involved themselves so wholeheartedly in Danielle's care and treatment. But her commitment to her child, which has been above and beyond anything else I have witnessed in the years I have been writing about medicine, must be put into perspective. For the fight, as Debbie seems to realize in relation to Danielle's upcoming education, is just barely beginning, according to Constance U. Battle, MD, Medical Director/Chief Executive Officer of the Hospital for Sick Children in Washington, D.C., professionally a national authority in the field of child health and development, and personally the mother of a twenty-year-old daughter with cerebral palsy.

In an article entitled "Beyond the Nursery Door: The Obligation to Survivors of Technology," published in the June 1987 issue of *Clinics in Perinatology*, Battle refers to a study conducted at George Washington University underlying the continuing stress on mothers with chronically ill respiratory-disabled children living regularly at home, a step Danielle and Debbie have yet to achieve.

"The most poignant aspect of the study," Battle writes, "concerns the multiple demands that were placed on ordinary people. They reported that their children and the delicate network of services that had been put together required constant vigilance. Even under the best-managed, best-insured circumstances, they were continuously concerned that nurses would not come as agreed, that equipment or supplies might not arrive as expected, or that some component of the daily plan would fall through. Their lives could become easily unraveled. Many mothers enjoyed no breaks, no evenings out, no vacations for years. The mothers felt that they had completely lost control over their lives and expected even greater problems in the future."

Battle also describes a dramatic and frustrating feeling of helplessness that she and her colleagues experienced during a presentation to the board of directors of the Coordinating Center for Home and Community Care, located near her hospital, by Angela C., the mother of an eighteen-month-old respiratory-dependent child living at home. "Like so many other mothers who care for these children, Angela appeared to be twenty-three going on fifty. She told us that she had rapidly matured and changed from a flighty teenager to an obsessive, mature young woman. Angela spoke frankly and freely of the stresses that have befallen her family and her concerns regarding the imminent birth of her second child.

"As board members, we basked in the satisfaction that the Coordinating Center had arranged home-care services and at least had minimized some of her stresses. And we did what altruistic professionals always do: we reinforced her heroism and applauded her martyrdom, but we could give her no answers for the future. We could not tell her how long nursing services would be provided or what would happen if [the state of] Maryland would not fund her services several years hence. We could not tell her whether there would be any kind of commitment to her and her child if the child reached adulthood. We could tell her only that we were glad that she had assumed the care of her child, as secretly we thought that she had absolved us of most of our responsibility for the time being and enabled us to put aside our own disquieting feelings."

Debbie Burdette's mission for her daughter's future may not seem practical according to the experts in public education who advocate "special" schools for "special" people, but five years ago other experts told Debbie Burdette that keeping Danielle alive more than a few days after birth was not only impractical but damn near impossible. So although she undoubtedly harbors her own deeply felt "disquieting feelings" about the long-range future of her daughter and the system in which she has placed her faith, Debbie has resolved to pay little attention to the experts and no heed to the odds against her success. She knows exactly what she wants to do, and if not how to *do* it, at least how to *begin* her unceasing crusade.

As we sat and talked in my office, you could sense that a plan was beginning to take shape behind Debbie's dark and steadfast eyes; you could almost feel the heat from the fire of her determination.

For a while she pondered a question I raised—the idea that Danielle might not survive on her own in an "alien" and to a certain extent "unfriendly" atmosphere, such as a public school. But then she replied, "If I am considered capable enough to take care of her at home, which I am—or even in the hospital—then I can just as easily take care of her at school. If they don't like the fact that I will be there visibly in the classroom with all the kids, then I'll stand outside at the window. I'll do whatever it takes." She took a deep breath and looked at Trish and me, just so we understood the extent of her deep commitment.

"I am going to make sure that my daughter gets to go to a normal school and that she gets the care that she needs while she is in that school. If she doesn't tolerate school, if she doesn't do well, okay, then she can prove that to me. Time will tell. But until she says that she cannot do it, until I believe that she cannot keep up, I will tell you this: I will not rest for one minute until I see Danielle in the proper atmosphere for learning. As long as I am alive and standing on my own two feet, I promise you, my daughter will get her rightful chance."

Index